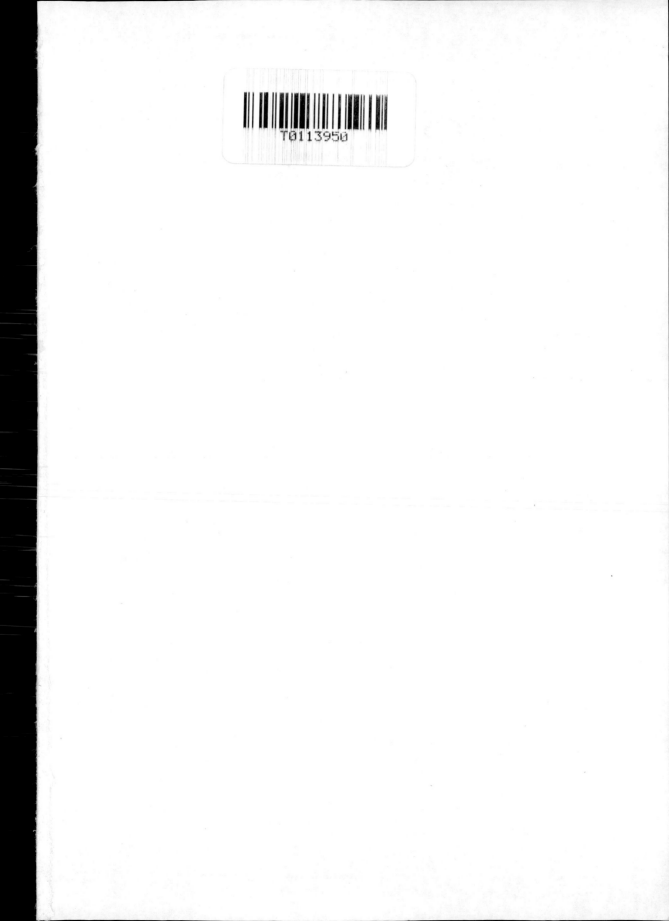

MEDICAL STATISTICS
FROM
GRAUNT TO FARR

MEDICAL STATISTICS
FROM
GRAUNT TO FARR

The Fitzpatrick Lectures
for the years 1941 and 1943, delivered at the
Royal College of Physicians of London
in February 1943

BY

MAJOR GREENWOOD
D.Sc., F.R.C.P., F.R.S.

Professor Emeritus of Epidemiology and Vital Statistics
in the University of London

CAMBRIDGE
AT THE UNIVERSITY PRESS
1948

CAMBRIDGE
UNIVERSITY PRESS

University Printing House, Cambridge CB2 8BS, United Kingdom

Published in the United States of America by Cambridge University Press, New York

Cambridge University Press is part of the University of Cambridge.

It furthers the University's mission by disseminating knowledge in the pursuit of education, learning and research at the highest international levels of excellence.

www.cambridge.org
Information on this title: www.cambridge.org/9781107652903

© Cambridge University Press 1948

First published 1948
First paperback edition 2014

A catalogue record for this publication is available from the British Library

ISBN 978-1-107-65290-3 Paperback

To

SIR ROBERT HUTCHISON, Bart., M.D., LL.D., D.Sc.

PRESIDENT OF THE ROYAL COLLEGE OF PHYSICIANS
1939–42

AN OLD FRIEND AND GRATEFUL PUPIL
AFFECTIONATELY DEDICATES
THIS SMALL BOOK

Est quadam prodire tenus, si non datur ultra

PREFACE

As said on a later page, when my lectures were written it seemed improbable that the Royal College of Physicians would care to listen to the briefest summary of them; so I gladly accepted the hospitality of brother statisticians and evacuated the lectures into statistical territory.*

The College, however, has resumed its normal activities and the editor of *Biometrika* has kindly permitted me to follow the practice of my predecessors and clothe the lectures in the form of a book; a small one, but still a book.

I have one, and only one, thing in common with the scholarly physicians who have lectured on Mrs Fitzpatrick's foundation. I have reached the time of life when looking backwards is more tempting than looking forwards and the sundial's warning:—'It is later than you think'—begins to have a personal significance. I look back with pleasure on the men whose works are slightly touched upon in these pages, my spiritual ancestors. They did not live very long ago; when the first of them was born the College of Physicians was more than a hundred years old. Their very names are unfamiliar to most physicians, their writings almost wholly unknown. I know I cannot make a ring of gold out of their little square, old, yellow books, only build a little cairn of stones in memory of them.

> What of it? 'Tis a figure, a symbol, say;
> A thing's sign; now for the thing signified.

M. G.

* These lectures were printed in *Biometrika* in three parts:
Vol. 32, Part 2 (1941), pp. 101–127;
Vol. 32, Parts 3 and 4 (1942), pp. 203–225;
Vol. 33, Part 1 (1943), pp. 1–24.

MEDICAL STATISTICS FROM GRAUNT TO FARR

By MAJOR GREENWOOD

INTRODUCTION

UNDER the Fitzpatrick Trust, a Fellow of the Royal College of Physicians of London is chosen annually by the President and Censors to deliver two lectures in the College on 'The History of Medicine'. I had the honour of being chosen for this office in 1940 but, for obvious reasons, the lectures were not delivered, and it may be safely assumed that some years will pass before a medical audience will have time to attend to the history of a subject the modern practice of which does not make a strong appeal to physicians.

The nature of the intended audience inclined me to stress the medical rather than the purely statistical aspects of the story and I have trodden ground over which a greater man passed some years ago. I hope that Karl Pearson's studies of some or all of these old heroes will eventually be printed, and I know that my slight essays can ill sustain a comparison. But, precisely because they are slight and linger over small traits and human oddities, they may, in these times, wile away an hour or two. I have eliminated some explanations which no statistician òr biometrician needs and the medical technicalities are few. Perhaps a note on the London College of Physicians as it was in the days to which these studies relate should be added.

The College was more than a century old when John Graunt was born, and the corporation consisted wholly of physicians who were Doctors of Medicine of Oxford or Cambridge; these were the *Fellows*. Physicians not Doctors of Medicine of Oxford or Cambridge were admissible only to the grade of *Licentiate*, and it was not until the nineteenth century, when Farr was a young man, that the exclusive privilege of the senior universities was abolished. It was not until Farr was a middle-aged man that the College had any direct contact with general practitioners of medicine and began to examine persons who did not seek to practise solely as physicians. In modern usage the College licence, L.R.C.P. (now only granted jointly with the membership of the Royal College of Surgeons, M.R.C.S.), is a diploma obtained by a large proportion of general medical practitioners in the South of England. Down to Farr's time, the L.R.C.P. was a 'specialist' diploma and could not have been taken by a general practitioner (the apothecary of those days) at all. The old L.R.C.P. is represented by the M.R.C.P. of our own time but with this distinction. Now, Fellows (F.R.C.P.) are normally chosen from the body of M.R.C.P.'s. In the past only Doctors of Medicine of Oxford or Cambridge could be Fellows, and before election but after examination were known as 'candidates', not licentiates. The great physician

Sydenham was never more than a licentiate. He graduated M.B. at Oxford and, for some unknown reason, never proceeded M.D. until near the end of his life, when he took the higher degree not at Oxford but at Cambridge.

I. THE LIVES OF PETTY AND GRAUNT

It is always rash to assign an absolute beginning to any form of intellectual effort, to say that this or that man was the very first to fashion some organon which has proved valuable. All we are justified in saying is that this or that man's work can be shown to have so directly influenced the thought of his contemporaries or successors that from his day the method he used has never been forgotten. It may be that the lost works of the school of the Empirics Galen despised anticipated the numerical method of Louis—some words of Celsus are consistent with the hypothesis. It may be that in the long succession of parish clerks who for more than a century transcribed the London Bills of Mortality, one or two suggested that these figures might have some other use than that of warning His Highness of the need to move into Clean Air. But we do not know. We do know that out of the casual intercourse of two Englishmen in the seventeenth century was produced a method of scientific investigation which has never ceased to be applied and has influenced for good or ill the thought of all mankind. In that sense at least we may fairly hold that John Graunt and William Petty were the pioneers not only of medical statistics and vital statistics but of the numerical method as applied to the phenomena of human society.

John Graunt and William Petty were both of Hampshire stock. Petty was of Hampshire birth, born on Monday, 26 May 1623, and was three years younger than John Graunt, who was born at the Seven Stars in Birchin Lane on 24 April 1620.

Materials for writing Petty's life are abundant; indeed a good biography of him was written nearly fifty years ago by his descendant Lord Edmond Fitzmaurice, and since then much of the material used by Lord Edmond has been printed. Sources for Graunt's biography are scanty, the most valuable John Aubrey's brief life of him.* Graunt and Petty became acquainted in or before 1650. The circumstances of that first acquaintance are interesting to those who meditate upon the perepeteia of human fate. It was the contact of client and patron.

John Graunt's early life and manhood were those of the Industrious Apprentice. His father was a city tradesman, who bred his son to the profession of haberdasher of small wares. John 'rose early in the morning to his study before shop-time' and learned Latin and French, but did not neglect his business. He was free of the Drapers' Company and went through the city offices as far as

---

* *Brief Lives, chiefly of Contemporaries*, set down by John Aubrey, between the years 1669 and 1696, edited by Andrew Clark, Oxford, 1896, **1**, 271 *et seq.*

common councilman; he was captain and then major of the trained bands (the ancestor of the Honourable Artillery Company). At the time of the Great Fire he is said to have been an opulent merchant. Even fifteen years earlier he—and no doubt his father (1592–1662)—had city influence. At that time a Gresham professorship was vacant and a young Dr Petty was anxious to obtain it. This young man's career had been unlike that of an industrious apprentice; it had been, even for the seventeenth century, romantic. His father was a clothier in Romsey, who 'did dye his owne cloathes' in a small way of business. When William was a child, 'his greatest delight was to be looking on the artificers— e.g. smyths, the watch-maker, carpenters, joyners etc.—and at twelve years old could have worked at any of these trades. Here he went to schoole, and learnt by 12 yeares a competent smattering of Latin, and was entred into Greek' (Aubrey, Clark's edition, 2, 140).

But the precocious lad did not find a patron in Romsey and was shipped for a cabin boy at the age of fourteen. His short sight earned him a taste of the rope's end, and after rather less than a year at sea he broke his leg and was set ashore in Caen to shift for himself. 'Le petit matelot anglois qui parle latin et grec' attracted sympathy and obtained instruction in Caen. Caen was not a famous seat of learning like Leyden or Montpellier, but the Fellows and licentiates of the College of Physicians admitted between 1640 and 1700 include the names of four persons who studied or graduated in Caen (Nicholas Lamy, Theophilus Garencières, John Peachi and Richard Griffiths). Petty, however, was not then thinking of medicine but mathematics and navigation and came home to join the navy. In what capacity he served is unknown; he merely says (in his Will) that his knowledge of arithmetic, geometry, astronomy conducing to navigation, etc., and his having been at the University of Caen, 'preferred me to the King's Navy where at the age of 20 years, I had gotten up about three score pounds, with as much mathematics as any of my age was known to have had'. His naval career was short, for in 1643 he was again on the continent. Here he wandered in the Netherlands and France and studied medicine or at least anatomy. He frequented the company of more eminent refugees, such as Pell and Hobbes, as well as that of the French mathematician Mersen. He was very poor and told Aubrey that he once lived for a week on three pennyworth of walnuts, but on his return to England the three score pounds had increased to seventy and he had also educated his brother Anthony.

At first Petty seems to have tried to make a living out of his father's business, but he soon went to London with a patented manifold letter writer and sundry other schemes of an educational character. These occupied him between 1643 and 1649 and made him acquainted with various men of science, among others Wallis and Wilkins, but were not remunerative, and in 1649 he migrated to Oxford.

Petty was created Doctor of Medicine on 7 March 1649 by virtue of a dispensation from the delegates (no doubt the parliamentary equivalent of the Royal Mandate of later and earlier times). He was also made a Fellow of Brasenose and had already been appointed deputy to the Professor of Anatomy. He was admitted a candidate of the College of Physicians in June 1650 (he was not elected a Fellow until 1655 and was admitted on 25 June 1658). At Oxford he became something of a popular hero by resuscitating (on 14 December 1651) an inefficiently hanged criminal, who, condemned for the murder of an illegitimate child, is said to have survived to be the mother of lawfully begotten offspring.

Academically Petty rose to be full Professor of Anatomy and Vice-Principal of Brasenose. It is at this point (as usual the precise dates are dubious) that he became a candidate for a Gresham professorship and made contact with John Graunt.

Although, as I have said, the materials for a biography of Petty are abundant, all we know of his early years comes from himself or from friends of later life who knew no more than he told them. We have no independent means of judging the extent of his culture. There is good evidence that he knew more Latin than most Fellows of the College of Physicians know now; none that he was an exact scholar (indeed we have his own word, which I am not prepared to gainsay,* to the contrary). He was certainly admitted to friendship by some men, such as Wallis and Pell, who were serious mathematicians, as by others, such as Hobbes, who were not. But whether he could fairly be called a mathematician is doubtful. Of his medical knowledge we know little. He left medical manuscripts, but these are still unpublished; of his clinical experience we know nothing.

Petty told Aubrey that 'he hath read but little, that is to say, not since 25 aetat., and is of Mr. Hobbes his mind, that had he read much, as some men have, he had not known as much as he does, nor should have made such discoveries and improvements'. But it is at least certain that he made a favourable impression upon men who had read a good deal and that the young Dr Petty of 1650 was thought a promising man. Still it *had* been an odd career and one wonders what a steady business man in the city of London thought of it.

Why the anatomy professor who had resuscitated half-hanged Ann Green should be made a professor of music is not obvious, and if the Gresham appointments were jobs, why should the job be done for Petty? The modern imaginative historian might suggest various reasons. For instance, that Petty made a

---

* If No. 88 of *The Petty Papers* (**2**, 36) is a typical example of Petty's Latin Prose style, there is not much to be said for it. Here is an example: 'An dulcius est humanae naturae permultos suam potestatem in unum quendam et in perpetuum transferre, id est pendis amittere quam ipso puel deindem servare, vel paulatium et in breve tempus irogare, a seipsis demo reformendam et disponendam alioquin pro ut, mutato tam rerum quam animi indies suaserit?' Some of the gibberish may be due to the editor's failure to decipher the handwriting, but no emendation could twist this into unbarbaric prose.

conquest of Graunt, perhaps had Hampshire friends who were friends of the Graunt family, perhaps talked about political arithmetic. We have no evidence at all. If the Gresham Professor of Music *had* duties, Petty did not perform them; about the time of his appointment he obtained leave of absence from Brasenose and within a year (in 1652) had left for Ireland, where he was to be very busy for some time to come and to make, or found, his material fortunes.

Macaulay (chap. III) says that at the end of the Stuart period the greatest estates in the kingdom very little exceeded twenty thousand a year.

The Duke of Ormond had twenty-two thousand a year. The Duke of Buckingham, before his extravagance had impaired his great property, had nineteen thousand six hundred a year. George Monk, Duke of Albemarle, who had been rewarded for his eminent services with immense grants of crown land, and who had been notorious both for covetousness and for parsimony, left fifteen thousand a year of real estate, and sixty thousand pounds in money, which probably yielded seven per cent. These three Dukes were supposed to be three of the very richest subjects in England.

In 1685 Petty made his Will. This Will is a curiously interesting document, because it is also an autobiography. It is rich in arithmetical statements and, like much of Petty's arithmetic, the statements may be optimistic. Petty's final casting of his accounts is in this fashion: 'Whereupon I say in gross, that my reall estate or income may be £6,500 per ann. my personall estate about £45,000, my bad and desparate debts, 30 thousand pounds, and the improvements may be £4000 per ann., in all £15,000 per ann. *ut supra*.'

The details of the calculation are perplexing enough; still if the above cited dukes *were* the richest subjects of the king and if (Macaulay) 'the average income of a temporal peer was estimated by the best informed persons, at about three thousand a year', Sir William Petty, of the year 1685, had travelled as far from the young Oxford professor of 1650 as that budding physician from the little English cabin boy who spoke Latin and Greek, in Caen, in 1638. The details of the fortune-building are not our concern. The shortest account is Petty's own in his Will. He says that by the end of his Oxford career he had a stock of four hundred pounds and received an advance of one hundred more on setting out for Ireland.

Upon the tenth of September, 1652, I landed att Waterford, in Ireland, Phisitian to the army, who had suppressed the Rebellion began in the year 1641, and to the Generall of the same, and the Head Quarters, at the rate of 20s. per diem, at which I continued, till June, 1659, gaining by my practice about £400 per annum, above the said sallary. About September, 1654, I, perceiving that the admeasurement of the lands forfeited by the forementioned Rebellion, and intended to regulate the satisfaction of the soldiers who had suppressed the same, was most insufficiently and absurdly managed, I obtained a contract, dated the 11th. of December, 1654, for making the said admeasurement, and by God's blessing so performed the same as that I gained about nine thousand pounds thereby, which with the £500 above mentioned, my sallary of 20s. per diem, the benefit of my practice, together with £600 given me for directing an after survey of the adventrs lands, and £800 more for 2 years sallary as Clerk of the Councell, raised me an estate of about thirteen thousand pounds in ready and reall money, at a time, when, without art, interest, or authority, men bought as much lands for 10s, in reall money as in this year, 1685, yield 10s. per ann. rent above his *Maties* quitt rents (*The Life of Sir William Petty*, by Lord Edmond Fitzmaurice, London 1895, p. 319).

No one would willingly rake over the embers of Irish history—still glowing after nearly three hundred years. Petty believed himself to be a good man struggling against adversity and a public benefactor treated with gross injustice to the day of his death. Lecky (*History of Ireland*, vol. 1, chap. 1, p. 111 of popular edition) took a less favourable view. Even if the subject were relevant to my undertaking, which it is not, I have not the training in historical research to justify me in writing about it. There are, however, some points of psychological interest.

Petty did not, like his contemporary Thomas Sydenham, actually take up arms against the king, but he was even more plainly a protégé of the king's enemies. Sydenham's military career was unimportant; there is no reason to believe that he ever exchanged a word with a member of the Cromwell family. Petty was the confidential adviser and close personal friend of Henry Cromwell; his services to the Commonwealth authorities were the foundation of his fortune. Like many people who have social gifts he had the gentle art of making enemies.

Pepys, Aubrey and Evelyn concur in the judgment that Petty was a most entertaining companion. Evelyn says he was a wonderful mimic. He could speak 'now like a grave orthodox divine; then falling into the Presbyterian way; then to Fanatical, to Quaker, to Monk, and to Friar and to Popish Priest'. The gift he exercised among his friends.

My Lord D. of Ormond once obtained it of him, and was almost ravished with admiration; but by and by he fell upon a serious reprimand of the faults and miscarriages of some Princes and Governors, which, though he named none, did so sensibly touch the Duke, who was then Lieutenant of Ireland, that he began to be very uneasy, and wished the spirit layed, which he had raised; for he was neither able to endure such truths, nor could but be delighted. At last he turned his discourse to a ridiculous subject, and come down from the joint-stool on which he had stood, but my lord would not have him preach any more (Evelyn).

My lord Duke was not the first or last person to fail to relish a joke against himself.

In *The Londoners* a challenged party names garden hoes as the weapons. That was Mr Robert Hichens's fun. In real life, Petty, challenged to mortal combat by a Cromwellian soldier, pleaded his myopia and demanded that the duel should take place in a cellar and the weapons be axes.

A man like this makes friends or at least admirers, also enemies. Long before the king enjoyed his own again, Petty had a host of enemies. When the king returned, one might have expected that Petty's position would be critical. According to his own account he *did* lose something, but he was knighted and the losses, such as they were, did not seem to stay the growth of his fortune. At the Restoration he was already prosperous and he died wealthy. Perhaps the explanation is that Petty was really as great a public benefactor as he thought he was. Perhaps the reason is personal. King Charles loved wits (in the old and new sense of the word) and Petty was a wit. The scanty specimens of what Petty's modern representative calls 'Rabelaisian' printed from the Petty papers would not have appealed to such a connoisseur in this genre as the king—we know from Halifax that the king liked to be the raconteur in this field and indeed repeated himself often—but he would have relished a good mimic. Still more important might have been their common virtuosity.

Charles was interested in experimental science, and although Petty certainly knew more than the king, he may not have known very much more. Neither Charles nor James would have been able to find more common ground with Isaac Newton than in a later age Bonaparte found with Laplace. But the ingenious Dr Petty, who had resuscitated half-hanged Ann Green (which would be a capital story if well told), invented an unsinkable ship, had a dozen plans for doubling the king's revenue, and knew something of everything, probably did more than Wilkins to interest the king in the new society of virtuosos (how the king must have relished the story of the planting of horns in Goa*), and he may incidentally have interested the king in his business affairs. This is all speculation; what is sure is that when Petty was back in London and able to renew personal intercourse with John Graunt, their relation was no longer that of client and patron. For a few years more, Graunt was to be a solid merchant, but before long Petty was the patron and Graunt the client.

At this point it will be convenient to conclude the biographical facts relating to Graunt. I take them mainly from Aubrey.

Graunt continued to be a prosperous city tradesman for many years after his first meeting with Petty. 'He was', says Aubrey, 'a man generally beloved; a faithful friend. Often chosen for his prudence and justice to be an arbitrator; and he was a great peace-maker. He had an excellent working head, and was facetious and fluent in his conversation.' Pepys thought as well of Graunt as did Aubrey, admiring both his conversation and his collection of prints—'the best collection of anything almost that ever I saw'.

From the Restoration for several years Graunt figures in London intellectual society (he was elected F.R.S. in 1663), but a material calamity was at hand. The Fire of 1666 no doubt caused Graunt direct financial loss; this might have been repaired. But, although brought up in Puritan ways, 'he fell', to quote Aubrey, 'to buying and reading of the best Socinian bookes, and for severall

* Sir Philiberto Vernatti, Resident in Batavia, had certain inquiries sent him by order of the Royal Society. The eighth question was: 'What ground there may be for that Relation, concerning Horns taking root, and growing about Goa?' This is Sir Philiberto's answer: 'Inquiring about this, a friend laughed, and told me it was a jeer put upon the Portugueso, because the women of Goa are counted much given to lechery' (Sprat's *History of the Royal Society of London*, 2nd ed. London 1702, p. 161).

years continued of that opinion. At least, about...he turned a Roman Catholique, of which religion he dyed a great zealot.'

Graunt's path to Rome was similar to that of young Edmund Gibbon, but the results on the career of a city tradesman in the days of Oates *triumphans* were more serious than a visit to Lausanne. Graunt became bankrupt. His name dropped out of the list of the Royal Society after 1666, and in 1674 he died. There is evidence that in these last years of worldly misfortune, when the wheel had come full circle since Graunt had secured the Gresham professorship for Petty, Petty helped Graunt. When Petty was in Ireland, Graunt acted in some sort as his London agent, and Petty conceived a plan of settling Graunt in Ireland. But (we have, of course, only Petty's word for this) Graunt was not an easy man to help; it is possible, of course, that he may have resented Petty's admonitions. 'You have done amiss in sundry particulars, which I need not mention because you yourself may easily conjecture my meanings. However we leave these things to God and be mindful of what is the sum of all religion, and of what is and ever was true religion all the world over.' This is an extract from a letter of January 1673 to Graunt (*The Petty-Southwell Correspondence*, p. xxix) printed by the late Marquis of Lansdowne. If Lord Lansdowne was right (the whole letter is not printed) in thinking this a reference to Graunt's conversion (or perversion) 'of which', says Lord Lansdowne, 'Petty seems to have disapproved on temporal rather than spiritual grounds', it might have hurt a sensitive man.

Graunt died on Easter Eve 1674 and was buried the Wednesday following in St Dunstan's church in Fleet Street. 'A great number of ingeniose persons attended him to his grave. Among others, with teares, was that ingeniose great virtuoso, Sir William Petty, his old and intimate acquaintance, who was sometime a student of Brasenose College.' Sir William outlived his friend thirteen years and lies in Romsey Abbey. Until a descendant in the nineteenth century (the third Marquis of Lansdowne) erected a monument, 'not even an inscription indicated that the founder of political economy lay in Rumsey Abbey' (Fitzmaurice, p. 315).

Graunt had a son who died in Persia and a daughter who, according to Aubrey, became a nun at Ghent. Nothing is known of descendants.

Petty's widow was raised to the peerage and her elder sons, Charles and Henry, died without issue. But the title was revived in favour of John Fitzmaurice, the second surviving son of Thomas Fitzmaurice, Earl of Kerry who, as his grandson remarked, had 'married luckily for me and mine, a very ugly woman who brought into his family whatever degree of sense may have appeared in it, or whatever wealth is likely to remain in it'. This ill-favoured woman was Petty's daughter Anne, to whom her father wrote:

> My pretty little Pusling and my daughter Ann
> That shall bee a countesse, if her pappa can.

The cynical grandson was George III's prime minister and afterwards his *bête noire*, 'The Jesuit of Berkley Square' and first Marquis of Lansdowne.

Of the two friends, one has left an intellectual monument only; descendants of the other have been famous in English history.

Of these, best known are the first and third Marquises of Lansdowne, William (1737–1805) and Henry (1780–1863). Of the first marquis, much better known as Lord Shelburne (the title created for Lady Petty), every schoolboy—not only Macaulay's schoolboy—has heard; the quarrel between Charles Fox and Shelburne, the party split, the coalition ministry and so on. Schoolboys who have reached the sixth and Lecky's *History of England in the Eighteenth Century*, know a little more. Shelburne, who had much more than a tincture of his great-grandfather's ability and applied himself to economic studies, was one of the earliest to appreciate the importance of Adam Smith and was highly thought of by two good judges of scientific ability, Benjamin Franklin and Jeremy Bentham.

As a public man, no parliamentary statesman before or since obtained so universal a dislike, a positive hatred shared by those who knew him and those who did not.

There is certainly nothing in the actions of Shelburne to justify this extreme unpopularity. Much of it was, I believe, simply due to an artificial, overstrained, and affectedly obsequious manner, but much also to certain faults of character, which it is not difficult to detect. Most of the portraits that were drawn of him concur in representing him as a harsh, cynical, and sarcastic judge of the motives of others; extremely suspicious; jealous and reserved in his dealings with his colleagues; accustomed to pursue tenaciously ends of his own, which he did not frankly communicate, and frequently passing from a language of great superciliousness and arrogance to a strain of profuse flattery (Lecky, 5, 136).

How far some of these characteristics may be recognized in Shelburne's ancestor, we shall inquire in due course.

The contrast between Malagrida* and his son Henry is shattering. It is *this* Marquis of Lansdowne of whom nearly everybody thinks when he sees the title in a book, and rightly so. Walter Bagehot wrote:

You may observe that when an ancient liberal, Lord John Russell, or any of the essential sect, has done anything very queer, the last thing you would imagine anybody would dream of doing, and is attacked for it, he always answers boldly, 'Lord Lansdowne said I *might*'; or if it is a ponderous day, the eloquence runs, 'A noble friend with whom I have had the inestimable advantage of being associated from the commencement (the infantile period I might say) of my political life, and to whose advice,' etc., etc., etc.—and a very cheerful existence it must be for 'my noble friend' to be expected to justify—(for they never say it except they have done something very odd)—and dignify every aberration. Still it must be a beautiful feeling to have a man like Lord John, to have a stiff, small man

* Malagrida was an Italian Jesuit settled in Portugal who was burned in 1761. The supposed jesuitical propensities of Shelburne led to the name becoming his popular title. Hence Goldsmith's unintended *mot*: 'Do you know that I never could conceive the reason why they call you Malagrida, for Malagrida was a very good sort of man.'

bowing down before you. And a good judge (Sydney Smith) certainly suggested the conferring of this authority. 'Why do they not talk over the virtues and excellencies of Lansdowne? There is no man who performs the duties of life better, or fills a high station in a more becoming manner. He is full of knowledge, and eager for its acquisition. His remarkable politeness is the result of good nature, regulated by good sense. He looks for talents and qualities among all ranks of men, and adds them to his stock of society, as a botanist does his plants; and while other aristocrats are yawning among stars and garters, Lansdowne is refreshing his soul with the fancy and genius which he has found in odd places, and gathered to the marbles and pictures of his palace. Then he is an honest politician, a wise statesman, and has a philosophic mind', etc., etc. Here is devotion for a carping critic; and who ever heard before of *bonhomie* in an idol? (Bagehot, *Works*, **2**, 64–5).

Of the father, Atticus (an alias of 'Junius') wrote:

> The Earl of Shelburne had initiated himself in business by carrying messages between the Earl of Bute and Mr. Fox, and was for some time a favourite with both. Before he was an ensign he thought himself fit to be a general, and to be a leading minister before he ever saw a public office. The life of this young man is a satire on mankind. The treachery which deserts a friend, might be a virtue compared to the fawning baseness which attaches itself to a declared enemy (*Letters of Junius*, Wade's edition, **2**, 248).

Naturally justice was no more to be expected in eighteenth-century newspaper diatribes than in the twentieth century, but a clever caricaturist does not represent Charles Fox as a living skeleton. Those who attacked the son—there were such people—took a different line, as Bagehot hints. Perhaps even in his very different character something of the ancestral Petty survives. We shall try to discover what this was.

Forty years ago Hull brought out an edition of Petty's tracts in which he included Graunt's work. In 1927 the fifth Marquis of Lansdowne printed a selection from the Petty papers and in 1928 the correspondence between Petty and his wife's cousin,* Sir Robert Southwell (*The Petty-Southwell Correspondence*, edited by the Marquis of Lansdowne, London 1928).

We shall have to examine in detail both the 'works' and the 'papers', but, as a light upon the character of Petty, the Southwell correspondence is the strongest we have. Southwell himself was some generations farther away from adventuring than Petty. He came of an 'undertaker' stock—the adventurers in Ireland of Queen Elizabeth's time—and his father was vice-admiral of Munster before him. He was born in 1635 (died in 1702), regularly educated (Queen's College, Oxford and Lincoln's Inn), knighted in 1665, for some time Clerk of the Privy Council, in the diplomatic service, held other offices, was a member of parliament and eventually settled in a country house near Bath. He was President of the Royal Society 1690–5. He might be described as a lesser William Temple; better educated and less selfish, not so able, but with the same cool, cautious judgment; a psychological antithesis of his correspondent.

---

* Petty married in 1667 Lady Fenton, widow of Sir Maurice Fenton and daughter of Sir Hardress Waller who, knighted in 1629, fought for the Parliament and was one of the King's judges; he was a major general in Ireland in 1650–1 and a patron of Petty there.

The correspondence covers the eleven years 1676–87. Both men were, even by modern standards, middle aged. They write one to another with complete frankness; there is a remarkable absence of the elaborate verbal formalities which in seventeenth-century and even eighteenth-century letters are so wearisome.

Petty's side of the correspondence consists roughly of domesticities 10 parts, eager accounts of his quarrels and law suits concerning money 40 parts, discussion of papers or projected papers 40 parts, add autobiographical boasting to make up the 100.

In the purely domestic part of the correspondence, Petty is seen as a kind, good-natured father interested in the doings of his relations by marriage, also as a very bad judge of others' feelings. I remember to have read an unpublished letter by the famous Edwin Chadwick, the great and very unpopular sanitarian of a century ago. It was written to a friend whose wife had just died of puerperal fever. Chadwick expressed regret in the shortest possible formula and assured his correspondent that the best solace he could have would be to assist in pushing forward a bill (which I think he enclosed) to promote some sanitary reform which would have the effect of making it less likely that other men would lose their wives in childbed. I remember thinking that, however sensible the recommendation, the man who gave it was not likely to bring much comfort to his friend.

Petty was very much like Chadwick here. Southwell lost his wife in 1681 and Petty condoled with him as follows:

When your good father dyed, I told you that hee was full of years and ripe fruit, and that you had no reason to wish him longer in the paines of this world. But I cannot use the same Argument in this Case for your Lady is taken away somewhat within half the ordinary age of Man and soon after you have been perfectly married to her; for I cannot believe your perfect union and assimulacon was made till many years after the Ceremonies at Kinsington.

What I have hitherto said tends to aggravate rather than mitigate your sorrow. But as the sun shining strongly upon burning Coles doth quench them, so perhaps the sadder Sentiments that I beget in you may extinguish those which now afflict you. The next Thing I shall say is, That when I myself married, I was scarce a year younger then you are now, and consequently do apprehend That you have a second Crop of Contentment and as much yet to come as ever I have had.

This remark, curiously enough, was not well received.

You doe not onely condole the great loss I have sustained in a wife, but you seeme to think it reparable.... But when by 19 yeares conversation I knew the greate vertues of her mind, and discover since her death a more secrett correspondence with Heaven in Acts of Pietye and devotion (which before I knew not of), you will allow me, at least for my Children's sake, to lament that they have too early lost their guide.

Petty could not, it seems, understand that Southwell was wounded and returned to the charge in a letter which is lost. That letter provoked a reply which even Petty could not misunderstand and elicited an apology (*Correspondence*, p. 90).

Petty was quite incorrigible. A few years later Southwell had another family bereavement and is condoled with in the following terms:

> That by the death of your Father, Mother and Sister, of Sir Edward Deering and your three nephews, you are the Head and Governor of both Familyes. That by the death of Rupe, Ingenious Neddy culminates; and by that of your Excellent Lady you are entitled to that million I mentioned of unmarried teeming Ladyes.

Once again, Southwell was not comforted. 'Cousin, you doe wipe off Teares at a very strange rate, but why did nature furnish Them if there must be no Sorrow?'

Petty had a very quick perception of when and where *his* shoe pinched, but no imaginative sympathy.

Passing to Petty's financial affairs and lawsuits, the position was this. By original grants, by purchase and in various ways, Petty had widely scattered Irish interests. Questions of the validity of the original grants, of rent charges due to the crown or to other grantees, of matters of fact and matters of law were endless. Petty saw himself steadily as a great public benefactor harassed by scoundrels, and it never occurred to him even as a theoretical possibility that others had rights. Of his manner of proceeding the editor of the correspondence gives a typical example (*Correspondence*, p. 90). In 1681 Petty gave evidence before Lord Chief Baron Hen as to 'Soldier's land' which he had bought in Kerry and, it seems, the court decided against him.

> Petty gave vent to his chagrin in a long and scurrilous lampoon against the offending judge, entitled: 'HENEALOGIE or the legend of Hen-Hene and Pen-Hene', in two parts. Whereof the first doth in 24 chapters of Raillery, contain the enchantements, metamorphoses and merry conceits relating to them. The second part contayning (in good earnest) the foolish, erroneous, absurd, malicious and ridiculous 'JUDGEMENTS of HEN-HENE'. Fortunately perhaps for the repute of its author, this diatribe was never made public.

Fortunately, also, for a more material reason; it would probably have led to a *second* incarceration for contempt of court.

Southwell evidently viewed his good cousin's proceedings with a mixture of gentlemanlike annoyance and practical minded contempt. He expressed these feelings more than once; the following extract from a letter of 1677 is typical; the particular suit in progress to which reference is made was a claim for £5000 in respect of a sum of £2500 actually advanced by Petty to the Farmers of Revenue.

> And suffer from me this expostulation, who wish your prosperity as much as any man living; and having opportunities to see and heare what the temper of the world is towards you, I cannot but wish you well in Port, or rather upon the firm Land, and to have very little or nothing at all left to the mercy and good will of others. For there is generally imbibed such an opinion and dread of your superiority and reach over other men in the wayes of dealing, that they hate what they feare, and find wayes to make him feare that is

feard. I doe the more freely open my soul to you in this matter, because tis not for the vitells that you contend, but for outward Limbs and accessions, without which you can subsist with Plenty and Honour. And therefore to throw what you have quite away, or at least to put it in dayly hazard onely to make it a little more than it is, Is what you would condemne a thousand times over in another. And you would not think the Reply sufficient that there was plain Right in the Cause and Justice of their side, for iniquities will abound and the world will never be reformed.

After all this is said, I mean not that you should relinquish the pursute of your 2500£, which is money out of your Pockett and for which you are a Debtor unto your Family. But for other pretensions, lett them goe for Heaven's Sake, as you would a hott coale out of your hand: and strive to retire to your home in this Place, where you had the respect of all, and as much quiet as could be in this life, before your medling with that pernicious business of the Farme.

There is no reason to suppose that Petty ever took such sensible advice. Yet, somehow, he kept his head well above water.

In the later part of the correspondence Petty indulges in that complacent financial retrospect which he inserted in his Will and I have, perhaps too harshly, described as autobiographical boasting. It is possible that Southwell had heard of these financial triumphs rather often; at least there is a hint of this in the following:

I will onely note that since you are soe Indulgent as to think me worthy of being your Depository in this great Audit, and expect by the Course of Nature that I should speake when you are Silent, you must allow me liberty without blame to aske questions when you seeme defitient or Redundant.

That you are defitient may be suggested when, on the fortunate syde, I find noe Item for my Lady or of the hopefull stock she has brought you (p. 227).

The shrewd thrust of the last sentence was deadly. The subject does not recur.

I have indicated the character of the non-scientific part of the correspondence because we must examine Petty's scientific writings in greater detail. I think, however, we have enough to justify a provisional diagnosis of Petty's psychological type.

In literature and in life the perennial boy is often encountered. But while Peter Pan and Mr Reginald Fortune make far more friends than foes, that is not so true of their living counterparts. The exuberant flow of ideas and schemes, the intense and restless interest in *everything* which is characteristic of the clever child, often is extraordinarily attractive when it is associated with and controlled by the trained intelligence of a man. But the bad as well as the good points of a childlike or adolescent soul* are to be brought into the account. The

---

* The first Marquis of Halifax said of King Charles that 'his inclinations to love were the effects of health and a good constitution, with as little mixture of the *seraphic* part as ever man had', and Petty held that the King was typical. In *The Petty Papers* (no. 93 of vol. 2) there is a memorandum headed 'Californian Marriages with the Reasons thereof'. 'In California', says Petty, '6 men were conjugerted to 6 women in order to beget many and well conditioned children, and for the greatest venereall pleasure, in manner following, viz.'

He then sets out the plan. One man 'excelling in strength, nimbleness, beauty, wit, courage

clever child is often naïvely and intensely selfish, and so remains as the eternal boy; his quite crude and unashamed egoism, his inability to understand that others have feelings and even rights, repel as strongly as his intellectual freshness attracts. How far he is a success in life depends on which way the balance turns.

Petty seems to me a good example of this psychological type; its good points, the restless energy and exuberant flow of ideas, were sources of strength in such a time as that of the Civil War and Restoration, which, particularly the Restoration period, was in virtues and vices an age of grown-up children. Indeed his emotional adolescence may have shielded him from the deadly enmity of real men. Its bad points made him enemies, but they were children like himself. Nearly a century later, in a time of adults, these same characteristics, restless intellectual energy and vanity, exhibited by one no longer a rollicking adventurer but a great landowner, produced an unfavourable balance and we have 'Malagrida'. In Malagrida's son, one has a change; the attractive traits, the eager interest in all sorts of things is still there, but the childish hungry vanity has been softened or sublimed. The cynic may say that it was easy for a great Whig lord 150 years ago to be agreeable, to keep himself *hors concours*; perhaps it was, although the *Dropmore Papers* raise doubts. The fact, however, is certain. In the third Lord Lansdowne one sees the good and in the first the bad effects of the perennial boyishness of the ancestor. The ancestor lived in a state of society where the good points outweighted the bad points. That is why, although he made enemies and was often vexed, he was able to view his career with complacency and to bequeath a great fortune. But it is not Petty as a man but Petty as a scientific worker who is the proper object of my study.

How far does the psychological make-up which, as I think, characterized Petty conduce to scientific investigation? We might expect that it would be an immense stimulus to pioneering, that such a man would direct attention to a number of problems which deserved study, but that it would not lead to the production of any solid contribution to knowledge. Our task is to examine in some detail Petty's scientific work.

and good sense' subsequently called the Hero, is allowed four women for his sole use. One Great Rich Woman is allowed five men who are to serve her when she pleases, but another woman is allotted to the five men for use in common by the five.

It may be said this fable is only an after dinner jest—perhaps that *is* the whole explanation. But Petty does go to the trouble of financial calculations, and does seem to suggest a serious consideration. ('The encrease of children will be great and good.' 'No controversy about joynture, dower, maintenance, portion etc.') Nobody emotionally adult would be likely to make Californian Marriages a basis for practical statecraft.

II. PETTY'S SCIENTIFIC WORK

It is no part of my undertaking to survey the whole of Petty's scientific activities, but to speak only of his medical and vital statistical work.

In Hull's edition of Petty's writings, the editor discusses Petty's status as an economist and remarks that Petty's view that value depended upon labour was probably derived from Hobbes. The corn rent of agricultural lands was in Petty's view determined by the excess of their produce over the expenses of cultivation, paid in corn, and the money value of the excess will be measured by the amount of silver which a miner, working for the same time as the cultivator of the corn land, will have left after meeting his expenses with a part of the silver he secures (Hull, p. lxxiii). Why there should be any surplus, he explains by density of population.

Prof. Hull refrained from attempting to assess Petty's work in terms of modern economic theory. A mere medical statistician will naturally follow this example. More than a century ago, Mr Chainmail had learned from Mr MacQuedy that the essence of a safe and economical currency was an interminable series of broken promises and added: 'There seems to be a difference among the learned as to the way in which the promises ought to be broken; but I am not deep enough in their casuistry to enter into such nice distinctions.' Medical statisticians may well adopt Mr Chainmail's modest attitude towards the whole field of economic theory. Confining ourselves to statistics, we must consider what Petty thought should be done and what he actually did himself.

Under the first heading, praise can be unstinted. More than 150 years before the establishment of the General Register Office, Petty specifically proposed the organization of a central statistical department the scope of which was wider than that of our existing General Register Office. It was to deal not only with births, marriages, burials, houses, the ages, sexes and occupations of the people, but with statistics of revenue, education and trade (see *The Petty Papers*, 1, 171–2). He did not confine himself to vague recommendations, but drew up an enumeration schedule to be used for each parish. On this was to be entered: The number of housekeepers and of houses; the number of hearths; the number of statute acres; the number of people by sex and in age groups, viz. under 10, between 10 and 70, over 70; for males those aged 16 to 60, and for females those between 16 and 48 and how many of these latter were married; how many persons were incurable impotents and how many lived upon alms. This, it will be noted, is a better enumeration schedule than any used in England before the census of 1821. Further in his notes (printed in *The Petty Papers*) are various suggestions for the utilization of data collected in this way.

The most striking is this: 'The numbers of people that are of every yeare old from one to 100, and the number of them that dye at every such yeare's age, do shew to how many yeare's value the life of any person of any age is equivalent and consequently makes a Par between the value of Estates for life and for years' (*The Petty Papers*, **1**, 193).

This is, I think, the most remarkable thing Petty ever wrote, for it *suggests* that he had grasped the principle of an accurate life table, viz. a survivorship table based upon a knowledge of rates or mortality in age groups. No such table was constructed from population data until the end of the eighteenth century, because until then data of the age distribution of the *living* population were not obtained. Whether Petty also realized that under certain conditions a life table could be constructed without knowledge of the ages of the living population is a controversial matter which I shall discuss later on.

Then he makes suggestions which are relevant enough to modern demographic problems.

> By the proportion between marriages and births, and of mothers to births, may be learnt what hindrance abortions and long suckling of children is to the speedier propagation of mankind; as also the difference of soyles and ayres to this foecundity of women.
>
> By the proportion between maryd and unmaryd teeming women, may be found in what number of yeeres the present stock of people may bee encreased to any number assigned answerable to the defect of the peopling of the nation for strength or trade.

There are not wanting some suggestions which imply that even if Petty's opinion of the Faculty were higher than that of Sydenham (whom we honoured *posthumously*) it was tinged with scepticism.

> Whether they [viz. fellows and licentiates of the College of Physicians] take as much medicine and remedies as the like number of any other society.
>
> Whether of 1000 patients to the best physicians, aged of any decade, there do not die as many as out of the inhabitants of places where there dwell no physicians.
>
> Whether of 100 sick of acute diseases who use physicians, as many die and in misery, as where no art is used, or only chance. (*The Petty Papers*, **2**, 169–70.)

This statistical experiment has not yet been performed and indeed might be hardly so conclusive as Petty implied.

When one passes from what Petty suggested to what he actually did himself, our praise must be qualified. As Prof. Hull said, he was 'more than once misled into fancying that his conclusions were accurate because their form was definite'.

In judging Petty it is but fair to contrast him with College contemporaries whose names are more honoured by us. Among his contemporaries in the College were Thomas Browne and Thomas Sydenham. Browne was a much older man than Petty, Sydenham almost his coeval. Of Browne's quality as a physician we know nothing; but his literary influence indirectly—through Samuel Johnson—and directly upon generations of readers has been greater than that of any other practising medical man. Browne, like Petty, had an enormous range of interests and his book learning was greater. But, as we shall see, when he tackles a problem of demography, Petty's rashest guesses seem by comparison as soberly scientific as an annual report of the Registrar-General.

Sydenham was an iconoclast in clinical practice and believed himself to be emancipated from the rule of ancient authority. No fantastic arithmetical calculations are to be found in *his* writings. In fact, with a single exception (*Observations Medicae*, **2**, i), no arithmetic at all. It never seems to have entered his mind, although his greatest work purports to give the history of the diseases in London through a generation, that the arithmetical statements of the London Bills of Mortality were of any value whatever.

Sydenham was too wise a man for us to think that he rejected the evidence because the data were compiled by illiterate old women. He would have known that the sworn searchers had the loquacity of their sex and rank and were likely to ask what 'the doctor said'. He rejected it, because counting and measuring things did not come within his purview, just as the first beginnings of pathology and medical chemistry seemed to him irrelevant.

For the most part, Petty's statistical work was severely practical, but there is one excursion into theory which is interesting. It is to be found in a section of his tract on the use of what he calls Duplicate Proportion and is reprinted by Hull (pp. 622–3).

Petty states that there are more persons living between the ages of 16 and 26 than in any other decade of life. The statement is not true for modern populations and was probably not true for the English population of Petty's time. In 1861–71 (before the fall in the birth rate and infant mortality rate) there were 5·4 millions living under 10, and 4·0 between 15 and 25). But perhaps Petty meant that there were more living in the decade 16 to 26 than in any *later* decade, in which case his statement was of course right unless the birth rate was falling.

He then asserts that the

Roots of every number of Men's Ages under 16 (whose Root is 4) compared with the said number 4, doth show the proportion of the likelyhood of such men reaching 70 years of Age. As for example: 'Tis 4 times more likely that one of 16 years old should live to 70, than a new born Babe. 'Tis three times more likely, that one of 9 years old should attain the age of 70, than the said infant. Moreover, 'tis twice as likely, that one of 16 should reach that Age, as that one of four years old should do it; and one third more likely, than for one of nine.

We have no life table for England in 1674. Perhaps the nearest modern experience might be the Liverpool Table calculated by Farr seventy years ago. According to that table the chance of a new-born child living to be 65 was 0·0976 and the chance of a person of 15 living to 65 was 0·202, which is about double the infant's chance, not four times as large. For the Healthy Districts, the chances are 0·4246 and 0·54585; that is, in a ratio of 1·28 to 1.

Petty's statements are wildly wrong. The interesting point is how did he reach them? The only figures he had were printed by Graunt.

This 'Life Table' gives l_x as follows:

l_0	100	l_{46}	10
l_6	64	l_{56}	6
l_{16}	40	l_{66}	3
l_{26}	25	l_{76}	1
l_{36}	16		

Now if we take 2 as the survivors to 70 (it does not of course matter what the numerator is for comparative purposes), then the infant's chance of surviving to 70 is 0·02 and the person of 16 has the chance $1/20 = 0·05$, a ratio of 2·5, not wildly different from the Liverpool Table figure and very different from 4·0.

A fortiori when Petty, having passed above age 16, asserts that 'it is five to four, that one of 26 years old will die before one of 16; and 6 to 5 that one of 36 will die before one of 26', we are in a region of pure fantasy because, even if he had had the statistical data, Petty would not have had the technical knowledge to solve the problem involved, viz. to find the probability that of two lives aged respectively x and y, the former will fall before the latter.

If we keep within the range of the simple arithmetic which Petty used, the result cannot be obtained.

He then passes to this statement:

> To prove all which I can produce the accompts of every Man, Woman, and Child, within a certain Parish of above 330 Souls; all which particular Ages being cast up, and added together, and the Sum divided by the whole number of Souls, made the Quotient between 15 and 16; which I call (if it be Constant or Uniform) the Age of that Parish, or *Numerus Index* of Longaevity there. Many of which Indexes for several times and places, would make a useful Scale of Salubrity for those places, and a better Judg of Ayers than the conjectural Notions we commonly read and talk of. And such a Scale the *King* might as easily make for all his Dominions, as I did for this one Parish.

The puzzle is to discover why Petty thought this statistical experiment proved his point and why he regarded the mean age of the population of a parish its index of longevity. The first question I cannot answer at all; about the second I can make a guess. *If* the parish population were supported solely by births and there was no migration, then, if the death rates at ages did not vary, the population would be a stationary population and both the mean age of the living and the mean age at death would be constant. The expectation of life is greater than the mean age of the living unless the rates of mortality at early ages are very high and the more favourable the rates of mortality the greater will be the difference. In Petty's day, when mortality at early ages was very high, the two constants were probably not far apart, but it is certain that both expectation of life and mean age of a life table population were greater than 16; probably of order 28 to 32.

I think we may be sure that the parish Petty counted was not stationary in the statistical sense, but had an excess of births over deaths, and that his average threw no light upon the rates of mortality.

Passing to practical statistics, it will be convenient first to note rapidly statistical observations which are incidental in treatises of primarily financial or economic interest. In the *Verbum sapienti*, which although not printed until 1691 was written as early as 1665, Petty attempts to reckon what a man is worth. Here is the method. He concludes from financial data that the annual proceed of the Stock or Wealth of the nation yields 15 millions, but that the expenses of the nation are 40 millions. So the balance of 25 millions must be derived from the labour of the people. He assumes that the population is 6 millions and that half of these can work, and earn £8. 6*s*. 8*d*. a head per annum. This would be 7*d*. a day, abating 52 Sundays and half as many other days for sickness, holidays, etc. 'Whereas the Stock of Kingdom, yielding but 15 Millions of proceed, is worth 250 Millions; then the People who yield 25, are worth 416 2/3 Millions. For although the Individuums of Mankind be reckoned at about 8 years purchase; the Species of them is worth as many as Land, being in its nature as perpetual, for ought we know.'

Why an individual's working life is worth only 8 years' purchase is not clear. One would be inclined to put it as the average number of years lived in the working period of life. Perhaps Petty took Graunt's table and worked out the average number of years of life lived between the ages of 16 and 56; it *is* nearly 8.

He then calculates the money loss due to 100,000 dying of the plague and makes it nearly 7 millions, adding that £70,000 would have been well disposed in preventing this 'centuple loss'. Perhaps this is the first printed statement of the neglected truth that public health measures pay.

Since Petty's day, others, including Farr himself, have done sums of this kind; it is a popular occupation in the United States of America.

Farr went to work more elaborately, making out a balance sheet of a man from the cradle to the grave. But the principle was much the same. We cannot say it is a *wholly* useless pastime. There is of course the difficulty that if more lives are saved the price of labour might fall. But to Petty that would have been no difficulty, because he held that wealth is *purely* relative, viz. that if the income of each person in a community is halved, everybody is as well off as before.

In the *Political Anatomy of Ireland*, Petty seeks to determine war losses in Ireland.

The number of the People being now *Anno* 1672 about 1,100,000 and *Anno* 1652 about 850 M. Because I conceive that 80 M. of them have in 20 years encreased by generation 70 M. by return of banished and expelled *English*; as also by the access of new ones, 80 M. of New *Scots*, and 20 M. of returned *Irish*, being all 250 M.

Now if it could be known what number of people were in *Ireland* Ann. 1641, then the difference between the said number, and 850, adding unto it the increase by generation in 11 years will shew the destruction of people made by the Wars, *viz*. by the Sword, Plague and Famine occasioned thereby.

I find by comparing superfluous and spare Oxen, Sheep, Butter and Beef that there was exported above 1/3 more *Ann*. 1664 than in 1641, which shews there were 1/3 more of people, *viz.* 1,466,000. Out of which Sum take what were left Ann. 1652, there will remain 616,000 destroyed by the Rebellion.

Whereas the present proportion of the *British* is as 3 to 11; But before the Wars the proportion was less, *viz.* as 2 to 11 and then it follows that the number of *British* slain in 11 years was 112 thousand Souls; of which I guess 2/3 to have perished by War, Plague and Famine. So as it follows that 37,000 were massacred in the first year of Tumults: So as those who think 154,000 were so destroyed, ought to review the grounds of their Opinions.

It follows also, that about 504 M. of the *Irish* perished, and were wasted by the Sword, Plague and Famine, Hardship and Banishment, between the 23 of *October* 1641 and the same day 1652. Wherefore those who say, That not 1/8 of them remained at the end of the Wars, must also review their opinions; there being by this Computation near 2/3 of them; which Opinion I also submit.

Assuming, which is rash, that the estimates of population in 1672 and 1652 are correct, the assumption that population varied inversely as exportation of cattle seems bold. Might it not be that shipping facilities were better in 1664 than in 1641? Had there been no exportation we could not infer the population to be infinite.

Again Petty has multiplied the estimate for 1672 by 1·333. But he needed the population of 1664, which presumably was smaller than that of 1672. If his estimate is right, the population was increasing at the rate of about 12·5 thousands per annum, so he should have multiplied 1,000,000 not 1,100,000 by 1·333 and has overestimated the 1641 population by 133,330, and therefore the number destroyed by the same amount, an overstatement of 20 %. But this is not all. If we assign the decrement of population between 1652 and 1641 wholly to sword, plague and famine, we must assume that births continued at the peace-time rate; not a likely assumption. Lastly, it seems unreasonable to assign the casualties to the two races in precise proportion to their estimated numerical strength in the population of 1641.

How it follows that 37,000 were massacred in the first year of tumults I do not know.

In a later work (*Treatise of Ireland*, Hull, pp. 610–11) Petty has another shot at this problem.

He now assumes that Graunt's deduction from a Hampshire parish register, *viz.* that christenings are to burials in the ratio of 5 to 4, applies to Ireland, and that the death rate is 1 in 30, i.e. about what Graunt estimated for London and much higher than his estimate for the country. He then proceeds in this way. He estimates the population of 1653 to be 900,000 and that of 1687, 1,300,000. Then taking 1/30 for the death rate and 1/24 for birth rate, he makes the population of 1652, 985,000. He does not comment on the great decrease between 1652 and 1653; but there was still war in Ireland in 1652.

He now says that the population of 1641 was greater than that of 1687, 'as appears by the Exportations, Importations, Tyths, Grist-Mills and the Judgment of Intelligent Persons'. This time he takes the population to be 1,400,000— a little less than in the earlier estimate—and by the same kind of reasoning again makes the war losses to be about 600,000. One is reminded of Hull's remark that Petty confused the accurate with the definite. Also one notes the inevitable tendency of a polemical writer—which Petty very decidedly was—to maintain his original assertion. Those of us who have *never* yielded to this temptation may cast stones at him. It is not I believe too cynical to say that *any* calculation Petty made would have produced war losses around 600,000.

Returning to the *Political Anatomy of Ireland*, we find here a distinct claim that the mean age at death (not the mean age of the living) measures longevity.

As to Longaevity, inquiry must be made into some good old Register of (suppose) 20 persons, who were all born and buried in the same Parish, and having cast up the time which they all lived as one man, the Total divided by 20 is the life of each one with another; which compared with the like Observation in several other places, will show the difference of Longaevity, due allowance being made for extraordinary contingencies and Epidemical Diseases happening respectively within the period of each Observation (p. 172).

Apart from what we should think the absurdity of basing important conclusions upon an average of 20—and Petty only gives 20 as a figure—the mean ages at death of different populations are not comparable unless in each place the population is stationary in the sense described above. But, since so acute a man as Edwin Chadwick made the same mistake in the nineteenth century as Petty in the seventeenth century and it continues to be made in various places in the twentieth century, we need not be superior.

We now come to Petty's purely statistical work which is concerned with the growth of population; before examining this in detail, it will be convenient to consider the methods available in the seventeenth century for estimating population and notions then current on what may be called the theory of population growth.

It is hard to believe that in the ancient world nobody studied demography arithmetically. There is evidence that the Romans enumerated citizens—the word census is pure Latin—and it has been suggested that the Romans made life tables. Gouraud, cited by Todhunter (*History of the Mathematical Theory of Probability*, p. 14), refers to a passage cited from Ulpian in the *Digest* which I have discussed elsewhere.* The question was of the value of annuities and the conclusion I reached was that Ulpian had no vital statistical basis whatever for his figures, that he simply began with the capital value the law gave for *any* usufruct and then, realizing that people do die eventually, made some subtractions, ending with the absurd (vital-statistically speaking) conclusion that after the age of 60 the rate of mortality was independent of age.

There is not, I think, any reason to believe that the practical Romans had anticipated Graunt and Petty.

That is not to say that nobody studied any demographical problems arithmetically. Indeed one Fellow of the College of Physicians who has had—and will

* *Journ. Roy. Stat. Soc.* 103 (1940), 246.

continue to have—a hundred readers for every one reader of Graunt and Petty, made an elaborate demographical calculation. This was Sir Thomas Browne. Sir Thomas devoted the sixth chapter of the sixth book of *Pseudodoxia* to the vulgar opinion that the earth was slenderly peopled before the Flood.

This vulgar opinion Sir Thomas found to be very wide of the mark. Indeed, far from the earth being slenderly peopled, 'we shall rather admire how the earth contained its inhabitants, than doubt its inhabitation: and might conceive the deluge not simply penall, but in some way also necessary, as many have conceived of translations, if *Adam* had not sinned, and the race of man had remained upon earth immortal'. Indeed Sir Thomas estimates that by the seventh century of the world's history its population amounted to 1,347,368,420. He reaches this result in the following way:

Having thus declared how powerfully the length of lives conduced unto populosity of those times, it will yet be easier acknowledged if we descend to particularities, and consider how many in seven hundred years might descend from one man; wherein considering the length of their dayes, we may conceive the greatest number to have been alive together. And this that no reasonable spirit may contradict, we will declare with manifest disadvantage; for whereas the duration of the world unto the flood was about 1,600 years, we will make our compute in less than half that time. Nor will we begin with the first man, but allow the earth to be provided of women fit for marriage the second or third first centuries; and will only take as granted, that they might beget children at sixty, and at an hundred years have twenty, allowing for that number forty years. Nor will we herein single out *Methuselah*, or account from the longest livers, but make choice of the shortest of any we find recorded in the Text, excepting *Enoch*: who after he had lived as many years as there be days in the year was translated at 365. And thus from one stock of seven hundred years, multiplying still by twenty, we shall find the product to be one thousand, three hundred forty seven millions, three hundred sixty eight thousand, four hundred and twenty.

	1.	20.
	2.	400.
	3.	8,000.
	4.	160,000.
Century.	5.	3,200,000.
	6.	64,000,000.
	7.	1,280,000,000.
		1,347,368,420.

Simply as a sum, there are difficulties about this result. If our 20 are equal numbers of males and females, it is not 20 which should be multiplied by 20 but 10. If they are all males, then women are left out of the reckoning. But, perhaps, as the Text does not record the ages of women, Sir Thomas esteemed them as ephemerids, sufficiently plentiful however to provide a wife for every husband. But then I think he should have said that the 20 to be begotten between 60 and 100 were all males. Anyhow the sum must be wrong because *some* of the 64,000,000 short-lived women of the sixth century should survive into the seventh Indeed Sir Thomas uses his data a trifle capriciously.

We must surely play a game according to the rules. We are to accept the

Text word for word as it stands. But, omitting Adam, whose age at his begetting of Cain is not recorded, and Noah, who seems to have reached middle age—500 years—before becoming a father, the reproductive habits of eight fathers are recorded. Two begat males at the age of 65, one at 70, one at 90, one at 105, one at 162, one at 182 and one at 187. When this primary business was over, they are all recorded to have begotten an unspecified number of sons and daughters. So, if we are to be faithful to the Text, a very much more complicated arithmetical problem presents itself. A male begets another male at an average age of about 100, he then begets males and females at an unspecified rate for say another 600 years, required the law of increase. The Text does *not* authorize Sir Thomas to start pre-diluvian breeding at 65 or to stop it at 100. His 'manifest disadvantage' is breaking the rules of the game.

Further, the Text does not entitle him to predicate of the other males the lengths of days and procreative exploits of the recorded eight.

All this, it may be said, is breaking a butterfly upon the wheel. Nobody now takes the statistics of the Authorized Version literally. The point is that Sir Thomas Browne *did*, but used them improperly. As Lord Chesterfield said to a Garter King at Arms of his day who had not followed the rules of heraldry, 'You foolish man, you don't know your own foolish business'.

Petty did not tackle pre-diluvian demography, but he did try his hand at an estimate of the world's population after the flood, 'To justify the *Scriptures* and all other good *Histories* concerning the *Number* of the People in Ancient Time' (p. 465).

As Petty was not going to allow the population of ancient times to be greater than in the seventeenth century, but to make it increase regularly from the time of Noah's Ark, common sense saved him from fantastic figures, but not from physiological difficulties. The rules of the game obliged him to start with eight landed from the Ark, so he thought it best to make them increase and multiply very fast indeed at first and progressively more slowly. At first he doubled the population every ten years, but by the birth of Christ has brought the period up to 1000 years. But doubling every ten years (in the first century from the Flood) leads one into difficulties.

We can allow the possibility of the four pairs emerged from the Ark producing 8 offspring in ten years and so becoming 16 in year 10, without too great difficulty. But ten years later they must number 32 and this *is* a difficulty. If the fecundity of the first settlers remains the same they will contribute 8 more children, giving us a population of 24, the balance of 8 must come from the four couples of children all of whom must be under 20, and this *is* a little difficult.

But at least we may say that there is nothing wholly fantastic in Petty's procedure. Petty does belong to a different arithmetical world from that of Browne. Here we may leave purely speculative demography.

To estimate the people of an area without counting them, we must count something which has a connexion with the number of the people. We may count the tax-payers, the houses, the burials, the christenings or the acreage under corn—all or any of these items vary with the number of people.

I wish to keep separate the discussions of Petty's and Graunt's statistical researches, but in the matter now to be examined Petty used some of Graunt's methods and results, so these must be considered.

Graunt used three methods of estimation. In the first place, he surmised that the number of child-bearing women in a community might be about double the number of annual births 'forasmuch as such women, one with another, have scarce more than one child in two years'. Then he surmised that families were twice as numerous as women of child-bearing age. His reasoning was that women between 16 and 76 might be twice as numerous as women between 16 and 40 or 20 and 44 (i.e. of child-bearing age), and he thought of a family as centred round a married couple. Finally, he thought that the average family would consist of eight persons, the husband and wife, three children and three servants or lodgers. So, starting with 12,000 christenings, which he thought a fair measure of annual births, he reaches 24,000 women of fertile age, then 48,000 families and lastly 384,000 persons.

It is quite certain that Graunt's estimate of an annual fertility rate of 500 per 1000 was an enormous overstatement. In London in 1851, the ratio of legitimate births to married women aged 15–45 was 251·8 per 1000. There is no reason to believe that nuptial fertility changed appreciably between 1660 and 1860. But an error of this kind would lead him to an understatement of families. Now, however, another error saves him. We cannot be so positive that eight to the family is a great overstatement as we can that the marital fertility was not 500 per 1000, but it is much higher than any nineteenth-century finding. Using *this* multiplier saves Graunt in this sense, that his quaint rule gives almost precisely the right answer for the population of London nearly 200 years after his time.

The legitimate births registered in London in 1851 were 75,097. This, according to Graunt's rule, is to be multiplied by 32. The result is 2,403,104. The enumerated population was 2,363,236; the conjecture is only 1·7 % out. *Sic me servavit Apollo.*

Graunt's next method was experimental and very briefly described. He counted the numbers of families in certain parishes within the walls and found that '3 out of 11 Families per annum have died'. He then multiplies the burials for the year (13,000) by 11/3, and proceeds as before.

Finally, he took Newcourt's map of London and

guessed that in 100 Yards square there might be about 54 Families, supposing every House to be 20 Foot in the front: for on two sides of the said square there will be 100 Yards of Housing in each, and in the two other sides 80 each; in all 360 Yards: that is 54 Families in each square, of which there are 220 within the Walls, making in all 11880 Families within the Walls. But forasmuch as there die within the Walls about 3200 per *Annum*, and in the whole 13,000, it follows that the Housing within the Walls is $\frac{1}{4}$ part of the whole, and consequently, that there are 47,520 Families in and about *London*, which agrees well enough with all my former computations (Hull, p. 385).

These conjectures led Graunt to think that the rate of mortality in London was about 1 in 32. In his first essay on the growth of London (pp. 458–75) Petty bases himself upon that estimate, and in the series of papers (pp. 505–44) this remains the fundamental method, but Petty allows himself to modify the multiplier, not altogether without suspicion of bias. At a quite early stage he had satisfied himself that London was the largest city in the world and much larger than Paris. This is the kind of argument. For the three years 1682–84, the average of burials in London was 22,337 and for Paris 19,887. So if the rates of mortality were the same, London was larger than Paris.* If the rate of mortality in Paris were higher than in London then the population of London must be larger still. According to Petty (*a*) a larger proportion of the Paris population died in hospital, (*b*) the mortality in hospital was heavier in Paris than in London. So it follows that the general death rate of Paris was higher.

That at *London* the *Hospitals* are better and more desirable than those of *Paris*, for that in the best at *Paris* there die 2 out of 15, whereas at *London* there die out of the worst scarce 2 of 16, and yet but a fiftieth part of the whole die out of the *Hospitals* at *London*, and 2/5 or 20 times that proportion die out of the *Paris Hospitals* which are of the same kind; that is to say, the number of those at *London* who chuse to lie sick in *Hospitals* rather than in their own Houses, are to the like People of *Paris* as one to twenty; which shows the greater Poverty or want of Means in the People of *Paris* than those of *London*. We infer from the premisses, viz. the dying scarce 2 of 16 out of the *London Hospitals*, and about 2 of 15 in the best of *Paris* (to say nothing of l'*hostel Dieu*) that either the *Physicians* and *Chirurgeons* of London are better than those of *Paris*, or that the *Air* of *London* is more wholesome (p. 508).

These, however, are only logical deductions if the user of the hospitals in London and Paris is identical. If, as implied in the first part of the quotation, we think of hospitals in the sense which our elder contemporaries think of the old-fashioned poor law infirmaries, viz. as refuges for the sick poor, it would mean that in Paris more of the aged indigent died in institutions than in London and heavy mortality might well have nothing to do with the skill or lack of skill of the medical staff. If we think of hospitals in the modern sense, then heavy mortality might be a mere reflection of the resort to these hospitals of persons suffering from illnesses which needed special treatment. In any case, Petty can hardly have it both ways. In another essay (pp. 510–11) he contrasts the higher ratio of deaths to admissions at l'hostel Dieu of Paris with that of la Charité, argues that the excess in l'hostel Dieu is unnecessary and proceeds to calculate

---

* It should be remembered that the London of Petty's calculations is the whole area within the Bills. The calculations of Graunt described above did not include Westminster or the six out-parishes of Surrey and Middlesex which were within the Bills: Islington, Lambeth, Stepney, Newington, Hackney, Redriff.

what the French nation would gain by saving this excess. But he has not in-quired whether the patients of the two institutions were *in pari materia*.

Here is an historical problem which might be solved by those familiar with the literature of the period. Its discussion would not be relevant here. It is, however, only just to Petty to say that, unless conditions deteriorated seriously in the following century, his strictures on l'hostel Dieu were justified. In Franklin's work (*La Vie Privée d'autrefois. L'Hygiène* (Paris 1890), pp. 177 *et seq.*) an appalling account of this hospital from the pen of the eminent surgeon Tenon, printed in 1788, is quoted. Tenon's description of the routine of this great hospital compares, unfavourably, with the story of the wounded in the Mesopotamian campaign which horrified England in the war of 1914–18. He remarks, *inter alia*, 'on ne guérissoit point de trépanés autrefois à l'Hôtel-Dieu, comme on n'en guérit pas encore aujourd'hui', and cites a court surgeon of the time of Louis XIV, i.e. a contemporary of Petty, to that effect. His account of the treatment of lying-in women is grotesquely horrible.

In another essay (pp. 533–6) Petty discusses methods of estimation more carefully than in his other papers.

He proposes to show that the population of London (within the Bills) in or about 1685 was approximately 696,000.

There are, he says, three methods: (1) From houses and families. (2) From an estimated death rate. (3) From the ratio of those who die of the plague to those who escape.

This last we may deal with at once. Petty asserts that Graunt had proved that one-fifth of the people died of the plague. But in 1665, 98,000 died of the plague; therefore the population was 490,000, and allowing an increase of one-third between 1665 and 1686 we reach 653,000.

Graunt could not have proved that one-fifth of the population died of the plague unless he knew what the population was, and he never claimed to have done so.

The other methods (which Graunt used) are rational.

To estimate houses, Petty used three methods. He says that in the Fire of 1666, 13,200 houses were burned and that deaths from these houses were one-fifth of total deaths, so he reckons the houses to have been 66,000. Then as burials in 1686 were to burials in 1666 as 4 to 3, he makes the houses of 1686, 88,000. He does not, however, say upon what basis the estimate of one-fifth of the deaths in 1666 stands.

Next, he gives an estimate of the houses in 1682 given him by those employed upon a map said to have been made in that year. This map has not been identified.

Lastly, he uses the return of hearths. In Dublin in 1685 the hearths were 29,325 and the houses 6400. In London the hearths were 388,000; so the houses on the Dublin ratio should be 87,000. In Bristol he says there were 5307 houses and 16,752 hearths, which give 123,000 houses for London; the mean of the calculations is 105,000. The Hearth Office itself, he says, certified the number to be 105,315. He must now have a multiplier. He accepts Graunt's multiplier of 8 as valid for tradesmen's families, but allows for smaller families among the poor and larger among the rich, finally choosing 6. He then allows for double families in houses by adding 10,531 to his 105,315, and multiplying the sum by 6 has 695,076 for the population.

Petty's second way was from an estimated death rate.

Petty multiplies the average of the burials in 1684 and 1685 (23,212) by 30, which makes the population 696,360.

He now essays to prove that the death rate in *London* was 1 in 30. He uses four arguments, of which only one is strictly to the point, viz. Graunt's direct observation that three deaths occur annually in eleven families—which however involves the assumption of eight persons to the families observed. Two others are relevant, viz. observations, apparently direct, that in 'healthful places' the mortality is 1 in 50 and in nine country parishes 1 in 37. The fourth partly rests upon a statement which Graunt did *not* make, viz. that one of 20 children under 10 dies annually. This fictitious value Petty averages with the statement of a M. Auzout to the effect that the rate of mortality of adults in *Rome* is 1 in 40. It will be clear that Petty has proved nothing at all. What he has done is to make it unlikely that the rate of mortality was less than 1 in 30. That, perhaps, was enough. One has a certain sympathy with his round statement: 'Till I see another round number, grounded upon many observations, nearer than 30, I hope to have done pretty well in multiplying our Burials by 30 to find the number of the People.'

With this I may conclude the analysis of Petty's statistical work. It will, I think, soon be clear enough that it is not of the calibre of Graunt's. Yet I cannot take leave of it without something of an *ave*. Careless, happy-go-lucky, tendentious; yes, all that. But anybody who has felt the exhilaration, to which Francis Galton owned, in the doing of sums concerning biological problems, feels his heart warmed by the arithmetical knight errant who had so many statistical adventures.

III. THE STATISTICAL WORK OF GRAUNT

John Graunt's contribution to our subject has always been regarded as one of the great classics of science. A few have indeed doubted whether so great a work could have been achieved by one whose material success was so modest and have sought to transfer the glory to Graunt's highly successful friend Petty. This dispute I relegate to an appendix. I assume that Graunt's published book is substantially his own original work.

The history of the material Graunt used has been written more than once and I have nothing to add to Prof. Hull's story. Graunt had, for a period of more than 60 years, arithmetical statements of the numbers of males and females christened and buried and of the causes of death (not distinguished by sex) under some sixty headings. He had no information as to the ages at death. He had no information as to the number or ages of the living population.

The first act of a scientific statistician is to assess the trustworthiness of his data, to criticize his sources. This tedious preliminary to the doing of sums was not much to Petty's taste. Petty, as we have seen, often used different data to reach some conclusion, but hardly ever discusses the reliabilies of the several data. Other Fellows of our College since Petty's day have made the same mistake. The terrible 'howler' committed by Dr William Heberden the younger, and detected, not without satisfaction, by Charles Creighton is classical.* But that was not a unique instance. Indeed, even trained statisticians sometimes confuse names with things. More than one rate of mortality has risen (or fallen) only on paper. Graunt made no such mistakes.

Graunt's *general* argument is that many causes of death are 'but matters of sense', for instance, whether a child were abortive or stillborn, and that in many cases the searchers are 'able to report the opinion of the physician, who was with the patient as they receive the same from the friends of the defunct'. But sometimes the searchers will be wrong and often enough the error will not matter.

As for consumptions, if the searchers do but truly report (as they may) whether the dead corpse were very lean and worn away, it matters not to many of our purposes whether the diseases were exactly the same, as physicians define it in their books. Moreover, in case a man of seventy-five years old died of a cough (of which had he been free, he might have possibly lived to ninety) I esteem it little error (as to many of our purposes) if this person be in the table of casualties, reckoned among the aged, and not placed under the title of coughs (348).†

No doubt this brutal common sense might set on edge the teeth of some Fellows of the College of Physicians even in the seventeenth century, but it was one of the qualities which made Graunt a pioneer. Making the best the enemy of the good is a sure way to hinder any statistical progress. The scientific purist, who will wait for medical statistics until they are nosologically exact, is no wiser than Horace's rustic waiting for the river to flow away.

Graunt, however, did not accept statements which he had the means of testing. Finding in a series of years that of more than a quarter of a million deaths only 392 were assigned to the Pox, he did not infer that Syphilis had been over-rated as a cause of death.

Forasmuch as by the ordinary discourse of the world it seems a great part of men have, at one time or other, had some species of this disease, I wondering why so few died of it,

* Creighton, *History of Epidemics in Britain*, 2, 747–8. Heberden supposed (erroneously) that 'Griping of the Guts' of the Bills was Dysentery and had decreased. It was Infantile Diarrhoea and had simply been transferred to the rubric 'Convulsions'.

† Numbers in brackets are page references to Prof. Hull's edition of *The Economic Writings of Sir William Petty together with the Observations upon the Bills of Mortality more probably by Captain John Graunt*, Cambridge, 1899.

especially because I could not take that to be so harmless, whereof so many complained very fiercely; upon enquiry, I found that those who died of it out of the hospitals (especially that of Kingsland, and the Lock in Southwark) were returned of ulcers and sores. And in brief, I found, that all mentioned to die of the French Pox were returned by the clerks of St Giles' and St Martin's in the Fields only, in which places I understood that most of the vilest and most miserable houses of uncleanness were: from whence I concluded, that only hated persons, and such, whose very noses were eaten off were reported by the searchers to have died of this too frequent malady (356).

In principle, the argument is still valid.

His next example of criticism is the case of Rickets, which first appeared in the Bills of Mortality in 1634 and then with 14 deaths only, but by 1659 had risen to 441. Was Rickets a 'new disease' or did an old disease receive, in the Bills, a new name?

To clear this difficulty out of the bills (for I dare venture on no deeper arguments) I enquired what other casualty before the year 1634, named in the Bills, was most like the rickets; and I found, not only by pretenders to know it, but also from other Bills, that livergrown was the nearest. For in some years I find livergrown, spleen, and rickets, put all together, by reason (as I conceive) of their likeness to each other. Hereupon I added the livergrowns of the year 1634, viz. 77, to the rickets of the same year, viz. 14, making in all 91; which total, as also the number 77 itself, I compared with the livergrowns of the precedent year 1635, viz. 82. All which showed me, that the rickets was a new disease over and above. Now, this being but a faint argument, I looked both forwards and backwards, and found that in the year 1629, when no rickets appeared there were but 94 livergrowns; and in the year 1636 there were 99 livergrowns, although there were also 50 of the rickets: only this is not to be denied, that when the rickets grew very numerous (as in the year 1660, viz. 521) then there appeared not above 15 of livergrown. In the year 1659 were 441 rickets and 8 livergrown; in the year 1658 were 476 rickets and 51 livergrown. Now though it be granted that these diseases were confounded in the judgment of the nurses, yet it is most certain that the livergrown did never but once, viz. anno 1630, exceed 100; whereas anno 1660, livergrown and rickets were 536. It is also to be observed, that the rickets were never more numerous than now, and that they are still increasing; for anno 1649, there were but 190, next year 260, next after that 329 and so forwards, with some little starting backwards in some years, until the year 1660, which produced the greatest of all (357-8).

This is an excellent statistical argument, and, incidentally, evidence that Graunt wrote his own book, for a physician would probably have suggested that the professional interest excited by the classical treatise of Glisson (assisted by Regimonter) which was published in 1650 might easily have increased the popularity of the diagnosis. Petty, who with Glisson, was a founder of the Royal Society, would hardly have ignored his colleague's work.

I cannot resist the desire to mention others which, while of little statistical importance, have a medical attraction. Graunt noticed that Stopping of the Stomach first appeared in the Bills of 1636, increased from 6 to 29 by 1647, by 1655 it reached 145, in 1657, 277 and 1660, 314. First he conjectured that Stopping of the Stomach might be the Green Sickness, 'forasmuch as I find few or none to have been returned upon that account, although many be visibly stained with it'. He thought that possibly Green Sickness might not appear in the Bills 'for since the world believes that marriage cures it, it may seem indeed a shame, that any maid should die uncured, when there are more males than females, that is, an overplus of husbands to all that can be wives'. Then he wondered whether Stopping of the Stomach might not be Mother, 'forasmuch I have heard of many troubled with Mother Fits (as they call them) although few returned to have died of them'. But he was diverted by guessing 'rather the Rising of the Lights might be it'. He remembered that some women troubled with the Mother fits did complain of a choking in their throats. 'Now, as I understand, it is more conceivable that the Lights or Lungs (which I have heard called the bellows of the body) not blowing, that is, neither venting out, nor taking in breath, might rather cause such a choking, than that the Mother should rise up thither, and do it. For methinks, when a woman is with child, there is a greater rising, and yet no such fits at all' (359). He notes that Rising of the Lights increased in the Bills from 44 in 1629 to 249 in 1660.

Finally, he suggests a correlation between Stopping of the Stomach, Rising of the Lights in adults and the Livergrown, Spleen and Rickets of children. 'And that what is the Rickets in children, may be the other in more grown bodies; for surely children which recover of the Rickets, may retain somewhat to cause what I have imagined: but of this let the learned physicians consider, as I presume they have' (359).

It might be suggested that one item under Stopping of the Stomach could be surgical, viz. strangulated hernia. Rupture was a heading in the Bills, but the numbers are small and show no regular increase with the increase of population. Graunt's attraction to what used to be called hysterical stigmata is interesting. One wonders how far these passages reflect conversations with Petty. It is clear that Graunt had no belief in the peripatetic uterus; Petty would have had none. The best medical opinion of the age is, of course, that of Sydenham. Sydenham (whose pathology was traditional) had a pneumatist aetiology of Hysteria, the origin was an ataxia of the animal spirits (which were the pneuma zotikon of ancient tradition). He not only believed that Hysteria might be a serious or even mortal complication of organic disease—as we do still—but that the ataxic spirits might themselves produce humoral corruption and lead to chlorosis or ovarian dropsy (*Dissertatio epistolaris*, 92). So there is nothing repugnant to the best professional opinion of the age in admitting Hysteria to the list of causes of death. Nor is there any gross absurdity in the suggested correlation of increasing Rickets and increasing Hysteria, from the point of view of a layman. But that surmise does not imply any professional hint, it rather suggests a belief in a merely physical factor, the pressure of an enlarged organ. That passage would not have been written by a physician.

These are sufficient instances of Graunt's criticism of sources—the temptation to go on quoting examples must be resisted. I pass to his great achievement, the estimation of rates of mortality at ages when the numbers and ages of the living were not recorded. For such an estimation to be correct, we all know that the population must be stationary, viz. non-increasing, not subject to migration and having constant rates of mortality in the several age groups.

It is a nice point whether Graunt or Petty appreciated the importance of these considerations. Graunt was certainly alive to the fact that the population of London was growing and that the growth was due to immigration from the country. The arithmetical position was this. In the earlier years of his series burials and christenings were about equal in numbers, in 1605 there were 5948 burials and 6504 christenings; in 1625, 7850 burials and 7682 christenings, in 1635, 10,651 burials and 10,034 christenings. Later the burials continued to increase, but the christenings either decreased or failed to increase in the same proportion. This Graunt attributed to neglect of christening owing to religious dissidence and gave excellent reasons for his view. It is clear then that there were two factors of increase, immigration and increasing numbers of births. Most of Graunt's deductions are based upon an analysis of the deaths by causes for twenty years, 1629–36 and 1647–58, which he selected as years comparatively unaffected by plague (of his total of 229,250 deaths only 16,000 were from plague).

If we treat this total as a denominator (or one-twentieth of it) it will, from the point of view of calculating mortality ratios, be affected by two errors. The deaths of immigrants will make it too large and the increasing births will make it too small. Can it be Graunt held that the errors balanced so that, arithmetically speaking, one might behave as if one were dealing with a stationary population? An alternative explanation is that Graunt did not realize the limitations of the method.

A third possibility is that, although he knew the fallacy, he believed that the incorrect method gave an approximation to truth sufficient for his purposes. This is the solution I should be inclined to adopt were I forced to choose.

As I have pointed out above, there is at least a suggestion that Petty did have some glimmering of the conditions to be fulfilled if a summation of deaths is to give a correct view of rates of mortality. I do not believe that Graunt was less informed on any point of vital statistics than Petty. However, all this is guess-work.

Graunt did not know the ages of the dead; what he did was to pick out of the list of causes of deaths those which he thought lighted only upon children 'not more than four or five years old'. He chose Thrush, Convulsions, Rickets, Teeth and Worms, Abortives, Chrysomes, Infants, Livergrown and Overlaid. These gave him some 70,000 out of some 229,000. Then he assigned half the deaths from Small Pox, Swine Pox, Measles and Worms without Convulsions also to children under six and reaches the final conclusion that about '36% of all quick conceptions die before six years old'.

Is this conclusion—I will not say correct, because we have no data to reach a correct result—but of a reasonable order of magnitude? The answer is that it is eminently reasonable. Two hundred years after Graunt's death, William Farr printed (in the famous Supplement to the 35*th Annual Report of the Registrar-General*, p. cxxxvi) an outline Life Table for London. This was, of course, computed by an approximately correct method, using knowledge of the numbers and ages of the living population, and reflects the conditions of seventy-five years ago. Interpolating in this we find that about 32 % of 'quick conceptions died before six years old'. There is no good medical reason for holding that the conditions of *child* life in London in the middle of Victoria's reign were much better than in the seventeenth century. The old genius used a bow with a frayed string and made no allowance for windage, but his arrow hit the target not far from the white. He gave the first quantitative measure of the Herodian sacrifice in towns, a sacrifice which was to continue to be offered for more than 200 years.

Graunt then passed to the other end of life and found that 7 % of the dead were 'aged'. He conceived that the searchers would mean by 'aged' persons of 70 years or upwards, 'for no man be said to die properly of Age who is much less'. His following suggestion that the proportion living beyond 70 might be used as a measure of healthfulness is not happy. But this calculation may have led him to make, or insert, the most famous passage in his book, viz. what is, in form, the first Life Table ever published.

> Whereas we have found, that of 100 quick Conceptions about 36 of them die before they be six years old, and that perhaps but one surviveth 76; we having seven decads between six and 76, we sought six mean proportional numbers between 64, the remainder, living at six years, and the one, which survives 76, and find that the numbers following are practically near enough to the truth; for men do not die in exact proportions, nor in fractions, from whence arise this Table following (386).

Graunt's figures are 100, 64, 40, 25, 16, 10, 6, 3, 1.

The one survivor to 76 is, as Graunt implies, a guess; perhaps he conjectured that his seven survivors beyond 70 died one a year. How he calculated his mean proportional numbers is unknown. Prof. Willcox conjectured that he experimented with multipliers of 5/8 and 2/3—the former nearly reproduces the figures (see Willcox, *Revue de l'Inst. Intern. de Statistique*, **5** (1937), 327). Ptoukha (*Congrès Intern. de la Population*; Démographie historique, p. 71, Paris, 1937) ingeniously suggests that he used the multiplier $(64-1)/100$ or 0.63.

We must, I fear, conclude sorrowfully that this shot did not find the bull's eye. If Graunt's survivors are compared with those shown in Halley's table (when correctly used, *vide infra*), for 100, 64, 40, 25, 16, 10, 6, 3, 1, we should have 100, 56, 50, 45, 38, 31, 22, 14, 6. It is possible that child mortality was lower in London than in Breslau, but quite incredible that later age mortality should have been so enormously higher.

But, of course, having regard to the data, it would have been more than genius, it would have been magic, had a correct result been obtained.

Prof. Willcox, whose opinion of Graunt is almost as high as mine, regards the passage as inserted on the recommendation of Petty and as Petty's composition. He thinks that it lacks Graunt's caution and suggests the flighty ingenuity of his friend. Prof. Willcox's arguments are weighty, but I am not convinced. That Graunt did not—to use the expressive slang—*feature* his table is true. It is also true (*vide supra*) that passages in Petty's undoubted writings imply that he had some conception of a survivorship table. But—and this is my main difficulty—if this were Petty's idea, I find it difficult to believe that he would not have exploited it. Halley, whose economic scent was not so keen as Petty's, saw the epoch-making importance of an idea which was to transform the business of selling annuities. It would be odd if Petty *had* seen it that he did not comment upon it. Graunt might well have hesitated, being a cautious statistician, but surely not Petty.

However, in spite of modern practice, the writing of history wholly in terms of psychology has its pitfalls.

Let us return to simpler applications of shop arithmetic. The advantages of country life over town life from the point of view of both mortality and morality had been a commonplace of poets, particularly those Roman poets who spent much of their lives in a city, long before the seventeenth century. Graunt was the first to apply an arithmetical test of mortality; he compared the statistics of Romsey with those of London. For Romsey he had ninety years' data of marriage, christenings and burials.

His statements about the population of the parish are not quite consistent. In one sentence he says that it 'both 90 years ago, and also now, consisted of about 2700', but a few lines later says 'it neither appears by the burials, christenings, or by the built of new housing, that the said parish is more populous now, than 90 years ago, by above two or 300 souls'. A little later he says 'it is clear that the said parish is increased about 300, and it is probable that 3 or four hundred more went to London; and it is known that about 400 went to New England, the Caribe Islands and Newfoundland within these last forty years' (389). Actually, from an estimate of the number of communicants (which he assumes to be rather more than half the total population) he makes the average population between 2700 and 2800. Taking the average of burials for the whole period to be 58, this gives him a death rate of a little more than one in 50, which he contrasts with the London figure of one in 32 (apparently based on his count of 11 families with 88 persons amongst whom 3 deaths occurred in a year; but this is a rate of one in 29).

There is no doubt a certain sketchiness about this, but it was not unreasonable to infer that the Romsey rate was much lower than the London rate.

Graunt found that, unlike London, Romsey had an average excess of christenings over burials, they were in the ratio of 5 to 4. He estimates that over the period the natural increase was 1059, and, as will be seen from the quotation made, he allots about a third of this respectively to London, to the colonies and to the parish itself. He argues that supposing the population of all England to be fourteen times that of London and other parishes to send one-third of their natural increase to London, then the London burials should increase about 200 per annum 'and will answer the increase we observe'.

Here again the argument is reasonable. He goes on to an investigation which has been severely criticized. He gives a table of the greatest and least number of burials in each of the ten-year periods for which he has data. In each decade but one the maximum is more than twice the minimum. But, he remarks, in no decade in the London experience is the largest number of burials twice the smallest number (he excludes deaths from plague from his statistics). 'Which shews, that the opener and freer airs are most subject both to the good and bad impressions, and that the fumes, steams and stenches of London do so medicate and impregnate the air about it, that it becomes capable of little more, as if the said fumes rising out of London met with, opposed and jostled backwards the influences falling from above, or resisted the incursion of the country airs' (392).

Prof. Hull shook his head over this passage. 'This is an attempt to explain by physical conditions the wide range in the observed country death rate which is really due to the narrowness of the field—a single market town—under investigation. It is perhaps the gravest statistical mistake that can be charged against Graunt' (lxxvii).

I do not like to leave a hero in the lurch. I must concede that if both Romsey and London burials were samples from a Poisson universe, the fact that the Poisson parameter for London was at least a hundred times that for Romsey would make it incredible that the London range, in terms of the mean or of the standard deviation, should be so wide as that for Romsey. But Prof. Hull was wrong in supposing that the wide range in the Romsey rates was due to the narrowness of the field of observation in a statistical sense.

Taking Graunt's 58 as the 'expected' annual deaths then, as 1/58 is small, the Poisson distribution is not far from the symmetry of a normal curve, and using the results of Tippett and E. S. Pearson, we may conclude that the expected range would be $23 \cdot 45 \pm 6 \cdot 073$. The observed ranges for the successive decades are 32, 48, 78, 23, 65, 39, 121, 91, 52. All but one is greater than the expectation and six diverge by more than three times the standard error.

Something more than small numbers is involved. Still, it must be confessed that Graunt did not anticipate the reasoning of James Bernoulli, although an intuition of genius may have led him to think that something more than 'chance' had play here.

Graunt devoted special attention to the demographic influence of the plague. In the first place, he remarks that the attribution plague understated the mortality due to plague. He infers this from the fact that in plague years burials from other causes exceeded the average greatly, 'from whence we may probably suspect, that about 1/4 part more died of the plague than are returned for such '. Next he inferred that after a great outburst plague lingered for several years.

> The plague of 1636 lasted twelve years, in eight whereof there died 2000 per annum one with another, and never under 300. The which shows that the contagion of the plague depends more upon the disposition of the air than upon the effluvia from the bodies of men. Which also we prove by the sudden jumps which the plague hath made, leaping in one week from 118 to 927; and back again from 993 to 258; and from thence again the very next week to 852. The which effects must surely be rather attributed to change of the air, than of the constitutions of men's bodies, otherwise than as this depends upon that (366).

Finally, he observes that within two years the city was re-peopled; a deduction from the time taken for the number of christenings to reach again the level of a pre-plague year.

We may, if we please, smile at Graunt's epidemiological inference. But it is a reasonable inference from the facts when we remember that in Graunt's day— in spite of Fracastorius—contagium was not thought of as contagium vivum, but as a mere sympathetic vibration or passing on of something.

I have, I hope, given an adequate sample of Graunt's quality, but have not mentioned the most famous of all his deductions. Both in London and the country, on the average more males were christened than females, but more males died young or entered celibate occupations. So we reach this conclusion:

> We have hitherto said, there are more males than females; we say next that the one exceed the other by about a thirteenth part. So that although more men die violent deaths than women, that is, more are slain in wars, killed by mischance, drowned at sea and die by the hand of justice; moreover more men go to colonies and travel into foreign parts than women; and lastly, more remain unmarried than of women as fellows of colleges, and apprentices above eighteen etc. yet the said thirteenth part difference bringeth the business but to such a pass, that every woman may have an husband, without the allowance of polygamy (375).

The story of how this arithmetical justification of God's providence attracted the attention of Derham, of how Derham's book fired the enthusiasm of the Prussian Army chaplain Johann Peter Süssmilch and of how Süssmilch's book influenced Malthus has been well told by Hull. I should not myself rank this section high among Graunt's researches. From a demographic point of view neither judicial hangings nor college fellowships could have had much effect in reducing the male excess.

Even copious quotation fails to convey the spirit of a complete book. I have quoted good things, but many more remain. Graunt revealed sundry important truths and not the least important was that very imperfect data, if patiently considered, will tell us something it is good for us to know. If young medical officers going to parts of the empire where organized medical and demographical information is at no higher a level than that of seventeenth-century England— and there are many such places—were restricted to a single book on statistics, I should advise them to take not a modern scientific work, but old John Graunt's *Observations*.

Did Graunt write the book published over his name?

John Graunt and William Petty were, as we have seen, close friends. Graunt, as the world judges success, failed and Petty succeeded. But by the judgment of scientific men in the seventeenth century, and ever since, the order of intellectual precedence was reversed. From the moment of publication a few discerning people perceived the originality and importance of the *Observations*, the same people who, while admiring Petty's verve, ingenuity and worldly success, did not take over-seriously his bright ideas.

But Graunt was a man of one book. Save a note upon the multiplication of carp and the growth of salmon, he published nothing more. Petty went on writing, scheming and talking for thirteen years after Graunt's death. That often enough in that period, the *Observations* were discussed over the wine—as they were quoted in Petty's writings—we may suppose. That Graunt discussed his work with Petty both before and after publication we may also take for certain, although we have no formal proof of it. The country statistics which Graunt first used were from Petty's native parish and even if we are not disposed—as certainly I am not—to give much weight to particular turns of phraseology, still there are sufficient verbal oddities in some pages of Graunt's book to suggest Petty's hand.

In these circumstances, it would not be very surprising if Petty's associates, particularly those who were not good judges of statistical work, were to conclude that Petty's share in the remarkable achievement of Graunt was greater than appeared. It is not even judging Petty too harshly to suppose that he himself might come to share the opinion. There is no evidence that Petty ever *did* explicitly claim the credit. In one list of his writings (one of four), found among Petty's Papers, he did include the *Observations*, which at least is evidence that he thought himself entitled to a share of the credit. We may suppose that if, in familiar intercourse, somebody had said 'Come, confess Sir William, yours was the hand that guided the pen of poor John Graunt', he might not have denied it very strenuously. I think I have produced evidence enough that Petty did not under-rate his powers and was not conspicuous for delicacy of feeling. My guess would be that long before his death he did come to believe that Graunt's intellectual success was due to his help.

Whether Petty believed this or not, it is certain that friends and associates of Petty began to believe it soon after Graunt's death, and the belief has been entertained by a few people in each generation since. These, with one conspicuous exception, have been drawn from Petty's friends or descendants or from literary critics.

In the seventeenth century, of Petty's circle, Evelyn, Southwell and Aubrey believed or said that Petty wrote or inspired Graunt's book. Two Fellows of the

Royal Society, Houghton and Halley, also attributed the book to Petty. The only one of the five who was certainly a competent judge of scientific merit was Halley. Halley began the memoir which contains his Breslau table with these words:

The contemplation of the mortality of mankind has, besides the moral, its physical and political uses, both which have some time since been most judiciously considered by the curious Sir William Petty, in his moral and political Observations upon the Bills of Mortality of London, owned by Captain John Graunt. And since in a like treatise on the Bills of Mortality of Dublin....But the deductions from those bills of mortality seemed even to their authors (*sic*) to be defective. (*Phil. Trans.* no. 196 (1693), p. 596.)

Since the seventeenth century, there has been unanimity among demographic statisticians and economists that Petty could not have written Graunt's book. Halley was quite as good a judge of scientific merit as any of them and a contemporary of the canvassed writers; if I were sure that he had read and compared Petty's acknowledged works with the *Observations* I should prefer his opinion to that of other 'experts'—including, of course, my own. Halley's direct testimony, in the sense of a court of law, would be valueless; he was only six years old when the *Observations* were published and became a Fellow of the Royal Society five years after the death of Graunt. There is no evidence that either before or after the period of writing and publishing his famous memoir, Halley worked on demography. After his memoir, but in his lifetime, a new epoch in mathematical vital statistics began. De Moivre, eleven years younger than Halley, brought out his principal works in the lifetime of Halley (1656–1742) and used Halley's table. The two men must have been well acquainted, for both were enthusiastic disciples and intimate friends of Newton, but Halley, like Graunt, made only one contribution to the literature of demography.

So it may be doubted whether Halley were sufficiently interested in demographic or economic writings to have read Petty's tracts at all. Also in the passage cited above (apart from the writing of 'authors' not 'author') the collocation of the *Observations* on the Dublin Bills with those on the London Bills is curious. There is no doubt that the *Observations* on the Dublin Bills were the work of Petty, and in the first edition of them they are stated on the title-page to be by the 'Observator on the London Bills of Mortality'. But this, as Prof. Hull pointed out (xlii), was probably a catch-penny device of the publisher, Mark Pardoe, to draw a public which had just taken a fifth edition of the London *Observations*. Actually the book did not sell, and when the publisher reissued an enlarged version, Petty's name appeared on the title-page without any reference to the London *Observations*. I conclude that Halley's evidence is less weighty than it seemed. He may well have had before him copies of Graunt's book and of the two editions of the Dublin *Observations*. Having no other knowledge of the literature he would naturally enough write as he did.

If we eliminate Halley, no other expert countenanced Petty's authorship and one, Augustus de Morgan, gave an amusing but quite cogent reason for dismissing the notion.

In speaking of the variations in the annual numbers of deaths attributed to Rickets, Graunt said:

Now, such back-starting seem to be universal in all things: for we do not only see in the progressive motion of wheels of watches, and in the rowing of boats, that there is a little starting or jerking backwards between every step forwards, but also (if I am not much deceived) there appeared the like in the motion of the moon, which in the long telescopes at Gresham College one may sensibly discern (358).

De Morgan (*Budget of Paradoxes*, 68; *Assurance Magazine*, 8, 167) commented on the improbability that 'that excellent machinist, Sir William Petty, who passed his day among the astronomers' would attribute to the motion of the moon in her orbit all the tremors which she gets from a shaky telescope.

Down to 1927 the matter was regarded, in scientific circles, as settled. In that year the late Marquis of Lansdowne published a copious selection of the Petty Papers with what he regarded as new evidence in favour of Petty.

The only new evidence of a direct kind was a manuscript list in Petty's hand of his writings or projected writings which included the *Observations*. There are three other lists which do not include the *Observations*, and if we are to suppose that the entry really referred to the book published under Graunt's name, then we must believe that in 1685 and in 1686 Petty had forgotten his best title to scientific immortality. The remainder of the evidence consists of parallel passages and *ad captandum* arguments to the effect that it was more probable that a physician had written on questions of medical statistics than a tradesman. This publication led to a lively controversy. Of the merits of this, I, as a party to it, am not an impartial judge. Purely literary arguments do not appeal to me when the question is of scientific method. Thus, Dr L. F. Powell attached weight to the fact that Dr Johnson in conversation had attributed to Petty an observation (not statistical) which is made not in Petty's writings but in Graunt's book.

In the discussion the word 'style' is used in different senses by the combatants. The statisticians are thinking of scientific method, the literary critics of verbal arrangement. To the former the fact that, particularly in the conclusions and the Appendix, Graunt's book has turns of phraseology which suggest Petty's hand, seems of little importance. To the latter it seems very significant.

In the article by Prof. Willcox, which I have quoted above, the controversy is reviewed, and the author concurs generally with his statistical predecessors.

Prof. Willcox does, however, differ from his predecessors in one important particular. He holds that the famous life table was supplied by Petty. He argues that this is far too conjectural to have been the work of so cautious a reasoner as Graunt:

In attempting to reconstruct its origin I have surmised that after Graunt had estimated that 36 per cent. of the deaths were due to children's diseases, that they all occurred under the age of six, and that the seven per cent. who were reported to have died 'aged' died at over 70 years of age (at one place he says over sixty), he felt unable to go further and reported his difficulty to Petty, already perhaps speculating about a series of similar problems.

Petty guessed at the number of survivors at the end of each decennial age period, 6–15, 16–25 etc. incidentally and characteristically ignoring Graunt's theory that seven per cent. survived seventy, and assuming instead, without reason, that one per cent. survived seventy-six and not one per cent. eighty-six, and that the survivors at age six decreased with each age period in a geometrical progression approximately equal to the 64 per cent. which Graunt had set for the first group (326–7).

Prof. Willcox's argument is cogent. It may be strengthened by a criticism of the late Prof. Westergaard (*Contributions to the History of Statistics* (London, 1932), p. 23). In using this table, Graunt made a serious blunder. In order to estimate the number of men of military age in London he subtracted the number alive at age 56 from the number alive at age 16. But this simply gives him the number *dying* between those ages; what he wanted was some average of the l_x's. It is evident that Graunt was not at all clear in his mind as to how to use a life table.

On the other hand, if this table were really Petty's idea, it is hard to understand why he did not exploit it. If Petty had been a Halley, the explanation would be obvious. The table is wrong; the conditions for the validity of the method were not fulfilled. There is indeed (*vide supra*) some evidence that Petty did know what data were necessary in order to construct a proper life table. One seems on the horns of a dilemma. If Petty thought the table was correct why did he make no further use of the method? If he thought it was wrong, would he have urged Graunt to insert it?

Although Prof. Willcox has certainly shaken my previous conviction, I still feel reluctant to surrender Graunt's table to Petty. However, there may be an element of sentimentality in this. At least the statisticians agree that the answer to the question which I have placed at the head of this Appendix is emphatically *yes*.

REFERENCES TO THE RECENT CONTROVERSY IN CHRONOLOGICAL ORDER

1927. LANSDOWNE, Marquis of. *The Petty Papers.*
1928. GREENWOOD, M. *J.R. Statist. Soc.* **91**, 79.
1928. LANSDOWNE, Marquis of. *The Petty Southwell Correspondence*, pp. xxiii–xxxii.
1932. LANSDOWNE, Marquis of. *The Times Literary Supplement*, 8 Sept.
1932. BRETT-JAMES, N. G. *The Times Literary Supplement*, 15 Sept.
1932. GREENWOOD, M. *The Times Literary Supplement*, 22 Sept.
1932. LANSDOWNE, Marquis of. *The Times Literary Supplement*, 13 Oct.
1932. POWELL, L. F. *The Times Literary Supplement*, 20 Oct.
1933. GREENWOOD, M. *J. R. Statist. Soc.* **96**, 76.
1937. WILLCOX, W. F. *Revue de l'Inst. Intern. de Statistique*, **5**, 321.

IV. HALLEY'S LIFE TABLE

The long and fruitful life of Edmund Halley (1656–1742) belongs to the general history of science; of him it may indeed be said *nihil quod tetigit non ornavit*. He made only one contribution to our subject, but it was of first-rate importance.

The circumstances of this undertaking are obscure; Halley would have perceived the imperfections of Graunt's life table, but it is not known whether it was he who set on foot a search for better statistical material than Graunt had had. Inquiries were however made, and made after he had become a Fellow of the Royal Society, so it is at least possible that Halley, who had travelled extensively in Europe (he was at Danzig in 1679 and in Italy in 1681), suggested that something might be found abroad. By 1691, the King's Librarian, Henry Justel, who was in touch with the Society, had been brought into communication, possibly through Leibniz, with Caspar Neumann, a scientifically minded evangelical pastor of Breslau. Neumann supplied the data which Halley used.

In 1883, J. Graetzer, a medical-statistical official of Breslau, published a little monograph* which throws light upon the work. He not only extracted from the Breslau archives all the data which were or might have been communicated to the Royal Society but had the Society's archives searched, with the result that a letter from Neumann to Justel and another from Neumann to Halley, both with statistical appendices, were discovered. Thanks to the labours of Graetzer and an essay by R. Böckh (*Bulletin de l'Inst. Intern. de Statistique*, **7** (1893), 1) we can form a reasonably clear idea of Halley's method, which was not what those who have not examined the literature suppose it to have been.

It is often stated that Halley, having found that during the five years of observation the number of births only slightly exceeded the number of burials, treated the population as stationary and constructed a life table by a simple summation of the deaths in the manner already explained. He was much wiser. What he tried to do was to construct a *population* table, in the following way. Suppose we know how many children were born in a calendar year, say 1690, in a town not subject to migration which maintains accurate registers of ages at death, and then we discover how many of the children born in 1690 will be alive on each successive first of January by a series of subtractions. We shall have the survivors on 1 January 1691 by subtracting those of the children born in 1690 who died in 1690. We shall have the survivors on 1 January 1692 by subtracting the deaths in 1691 occurring among the survivors to 1 January 1691, and so on. This will give a precise enumeration of the living population, and this is what Halley wanted. The figures we shall obtain will *not* be the conventional l_x's of a Life or (as German writers say) Mortality Table, but what in most modern books are represented by the capital letter L or years of life lived or

---

* Graetzer, J., *Edmund Halley und Caspar Neumann*, 1883.

'persons' living between the termini (see Appendix). *If* the population is stationary, the sum of these figures gives the population of the place under study. Now for ages between 1 (last birthday) and very advanced ages, L_x is simply l_x diminished by $\frac{1}{2}(l_x - l_{x+1})$. In the first year of life (and at advanced ages) the difference is greater. Thus in the first year of life deaths are not evenly distributed throughout the year of life, more than 70% of them occur in the first six months of life, so that instead of subtracting half the deaths we must subtract nearly three-quarters. Halley himself assigned 68% of deaths in the first year of life to the first half of the first year. The reason why Halley proceeded in this way was that he knew the population *not* to be stationary. His idea was to obtain the figures for the first few years of life accurately—indeed just as they are now obtained—and then to correct for excess of births over deaths.

His masterly plan was partly defeated by the fact that his Breslau correspondent Neumann was not so good a statistician as he was. Halley's letter to Neumann has not been preserved, we have only Neumann's answer of 1 March 1694. Probably Halley asked Neumann to send him (as a check on the calculations he had already made) the exact numbers of survivors on 1 January for five years, of births in a calendar year. Neumann did send him a table, but the table, as Graetzer pointed out, is wrong. Neumann gave the correct figures for 1 January of the first successive year, incorrect figures for the other years. Between 1 January of the year following the year the births of which are under study, and the next first of January, some of those born in the starting year will die under and some over a year of age. Neumann merely deducted the former, so he has too many survivors. To reach the right figure would have meant taking more trouble and he did not appreciate the importance of this. Böckh—whose opinion of his statistical contemporaries has a tinge of bitterness rare, of course, in other scientific pursuits—remarks that it was not strange Neumann should miss the point as it had been missed by many statisticians long after his time. It is at least clear that Halley had realized an important truth which did not become part of even expert knowledge for more than a century.

The precise arithmetical details of Halley's work are not perhaps of much medical interest. Graetzer and Böckh have done a good deal to clear it up. The data used (an average of five years) had 1238 births and 1174 deaths and the table accounts for 1238 deaths. Halley must therefore have had a plan for increasing deaths. It is likely, from an observation he makes on mortality in Christ's Hospital, that he did not *wholly* depend on the Breslau figures. Graetzer suggests that Halley may have made two graphs, one having an ordinate of 1238 at the origin and an ordinate of 64 at the oldest age, the other an ordinate of 1174 at the origin and 0 at the oldest age and that he plotted the survivors for each graph based on recorded deaths and drew a curve passing through 1238 and 0 between these graphs. It may be so. Using the original material which Graetzer published, Böckh recalculated the table. The results do not, except at ages over 60, differ materially from Halley's. So far as concerns the mean after life time (expectation of life), Halley's table gives 27·54 years at birth, Graetzer's material 27·69. For ages under 40 the re-working gives slightly lower and for later ages higher mortality. It may be noted that Halley's table gives appreciably *higher* mortality in childhood than Graunt's, more than 43% instead of 36% are dead by the age of six years. But Graunt's method would exaggerate mortality (so would Halley's method, but, owing to his precautions, not so greatly). On the other hand, Graunt's estimate of age is only an intelligent guess. Actually, as Graetzer showed, the infant and child mortality shown by Halley's table differed little from the observed rates of mortality in the city of Breslau in 1876–80.

It has been said that Halley was not greatly interested in the medical aspects of his work. After describing methods of calculating the prices of annuities, he has the following passage*:

> It may be objected that the different salubrity of places does hinder this proposal from being universal; nor can it be denied. But by the number that die being 1,174 per annum in 34,000 it does appear that about a 30th. part die yearly as Sir William Petty has computed for London; and the number that die in infancy is a good argument that the air is but indifferently salubrious. So that by what I can learn, there cannot perhaps be one better place proposed for a standard. At least 'tis desired, that in imitation hereof the curious in other cities would attempt something of the same nature, than which nothing perhaps can be more useful.

That the mortality of childhood depends upon the atmosphere is not so foolish an hypothesis as it may seem to us. Halley lived before breast-feeding became the exception rather than the rule. The 'curious' in other cities had not the wit to follow his advice. He made no other contribution to the science of vital statistics; a gain to astronomy but a heavy loss to demography.

APPENDIX

Halley's table is printed in two columns, the first headed 'Age current', the second 'Persons'. Thus:

Age current	Persons
1	1000
2	855
3	798
4	760
5	732
6	710
7	692
8	680
9	670
10	661

and so on.

* I have read Halley's paper in the collection of papers, many by him, collected under the title *Miscellanea Curiosa*, printed in London in 1705; the quotation is from p. 300.

A mistake sometimes made is to suppose that Halley meant by age current simply the end of each year of life and that the entry against each 'age current' is the number of survivors at exact age one year less than the 'age current', viz. that of 1000 born 855 survived to the first anniversary, 798 to the second anniversary, etc. The fact that Halley uses the round number 1000 for a first entry does something to encourage the mistake among readers who have not consulted the original paper and it is sometimes made by people who should know better. It is actually a terrible 'howler', leading to a wholly false view of rates of mortality in early life. Thus if 1000 and 855 were really the first two entries of a Life Table as set out now, then, as the first two entries in English Life Table no. 7 Males (mortality 1901–10) are 1000 and 856, we might conclude that mortality in the first year of life was no lower in 1901–10 than in Breslau in the last years of the seventeenth century. But the 1000 of Halley's table is *not* the number of new-born children but the average number out of 1238 born living between the ages of 0 and 1. This is what is called the L_x of a modern table or the population living between the ages x and $x + 1$. If we have a column of L_x's, which is what Halley gives us, we can deduce therefrom the more familiar l_x's provided we know the starting value and the number of deaths in the first year of life. Halley gives both items. He says that of 1238 annual births 348 die annually. So that his l_0 is not 1000 but 1238, and his l_1 is 890. He chose 1000 for L_0 by assuming that of the 348 deaths in the first year of life 238 occurred in the first six months of life, 68 %. This differs very little from the modern practice; in Life Table no. 7 quoted above 73·5 % of the deaths in the first year of life are assigned to the first six months of life. Having been given l_0 and l_1 we can deduce the other l's from the values of the L's which Halley gives because, after the end of the first year of life there is little error in supposing that the deaths between two birthdays are evenly distributed over the year; so, for instance, l_2 will be equal to L_1 less half the difference between l_1 and l_2, and proceeding in this way we put Halley's table into modern form. I attach a table calculated by Böckh.

It will be seen that, if Halley's table is properly used, the comparison is not of 1000 and 855 with 1000 and 856 but of 1000 and 719 with 1000 and 856.

Actually this is still slightly optimistic, because I am comparing 'persons' with males. The 'persons' figure for 1901–10 is 1000, 869. On the other hand, in the Breslau data still births (or some of them) are included in births, so that the mortality is slightly exaggerated. If for instance 7 % are still born, the survivors to 1 will be the same, but the l_0 should be reduced to 930. Or alternatively we should write 1000 and 773.

I attach Halley's table reduced to modern form and with the corresponding expectations of life calculated by Böckh (I have reworked some of the values from the data and agree with Böckh's figures).

Halley's Table, expressed in modern form together with the Expectations of Life
at quinquennial intervals (Böckh)

Age	l_x	$\mathring{e}_x$	Age	l_x	$\mathring{e}_x$
0	10,000	27·54	40	3,557	22·05
5	5,816	41·47	45	3,167	19·47
10	5,307	40·25	50	2,751	17·05
15	5,049	37·19	55	2,319	14·75
20	4,806	33·93	60	1,914	12·33
25	4,552	30·69	65	1,511	9·96
30	4,257	27·64	70	1,103	7·74
35	3,921	24·78	75	670	7·50

V. GUESSING THE POPULATION

My object is to trace the growth in our country of that part of statistical science which is of interest to students of medicine or public health. In speaking of such pioneers as Graunt, Petty and Halley it was proper to construe the obligation rather freely. Both Graunt and Petty did clearly perceive the relevance of their researches to matters of public health or even clinical medicine, but much of what Petty did had a more direct bearing upon political questions than those of public health. Again, the life table is a way of expressing the facts of mortality which is valuable in some medical researches, but its importance as a statistical instrument has been much greater in non-medical than medical circles, above all of course in the financing of assurance business. The commercial importance of life tables was perceived by Halley and by other mathematicians of his and the following generations.

Looking at the position after Halley's publication it was clear that progress might be made (1) in improving the accuracy of the life table, viz. by obtaining data more relevant to the conditions of life of persons who assured their lives or bought annuities, (2) in simplifying the very laborious calculations which the determination of praemia or purchase values required. Under (1) no progress worth speaking of was made in England until the end of the eighteenth century. This was partly due, as we shall see, to a not entirely unjustified disbelief in the powers of the medical profession to change the rate of mortality, partly to ignorance. No first-rate English mathematician after Halley gave any critical attention to the theory of the Life Table before the nineteenth century. Under (2) considerable progress was made, but this progress is of little or no medical interest and to describe it would involve entering upon tedious arithmetical and algebraical detail. The primary medical-statistical quaesita are correct enumerations of deaths by sex at ages and by causes, and of the numbers living in sex and age groups. When these have been satisfied, the medical statistician can get to work.

For 150 years after Graunt's death very little was done to improve matters. Down to 1801 the population as a whole had not been counted; forty years more passed before a reasonable age distribution was secured, and it was thirty-eight years after the first denominator (populations) that the first numerator (deaths) of the fundamental fractions was obtained. Until 1801 intelligent guessing was the method and the guesses of the eighteenth century deserve a few pages, if only because they prove that statistical ability is as rare as other kinds of ability and that wishful thinking is not a modern foible.

The first estimator to mention belongs to the seventeenth century and was a younger contemporary of Graunt and Petty, Gregory King (1648–1712). He was born in Lichfield, the son of a land surveyor. At the age of fourteen he was recommended as a clerk to the famous herald Dugdale with whom he worked for several years; after Dugdale had finished his Visitation, King worked for various amateur antiquaries and was eventually invited by a lady of property in Sandon (Staffordshire) to be her steward, auditor and secretary. Here he remained until 1672 when he moved to London and, no doubt through Dugdale's recommendation, had a considerable amount of employment in both heraldic work and ordinary surveying. In 1677 he became a member of the College of Arms, in which he attained the rank of Lancaster Herald and so continued until his death, but worked for other official bodies on financial subjects.

. The decorous memoir by George Chalmers, from which I have extracted these particulars, does not give us a very life-like picture of the man himself. There is a certain likeness between the early careers of Petty and King. King was not indeed shipped as a cabin boy, but Mr King (the elder) drank (if we may venture so coarse an abbreviation of Chalmers's statement that the father studied and practised his profession 'with more attention to good fellowship than mathematical studies generally allow') and King junior was a pupil teacher at eleven. If he really read Hesiod and Homer, made Greek verses and taught himself to survey land in his thirteenth year he must have had Petty's precocity. Both Petty and King had experience of practical surveying and, of course, both were interested in political arithmetic. But there the parallel ends. King was a professional surveyor and archivist and had a reasonably successful professional career. Petty was—Petty. One might, perhaps, adduce as another parallel that King made some enemies and thought himself ill-used. But the job by which Sir John Vanbrugh, a stranger to the College of Arms, was made a king-at-arms over the head of an official of twenty years' standing would have galled the meekest of mankind. One may safely conclude that King had more knowledge of the data of political arithmetic than Petty and less originality. His vital statistical work was not published until nearly a century after his death, as an appendix to the second edition of *An Estimate of the Comparative Strength of Great Britain* by George Chalmers, London, 1803. Perhaps he never intended to publish it—he communicated the substance to his contemporary Davenant—

and this may explain why there are no details of how some of his results were reached. The report reads rather like a document prepared for official use by persons interested in results not methods.

The starting-point of King's attempt to estimate the population was a return from the Hearth Office of the number of houses assessed to tax on Lady Day, 1690. That was 1,319,215 which, King estimated, had increased to 1,326,000 by 1695. He deducted 30,000 for empty divided houses,* took the round figure of 1,300,000 and assigned 105,000 to the London area, 195,000 to other cities and market towns and 1,000,000 to villages and hamlets. He used a series of multipliers, 5·4 for a house within the walls of London, 4·6 for a house within the liberties, 4·4 for the out parishes in Surrey and Middlesex and 4·3 for Westminster. For other towns, his multiplier was 4·3 and for villages 4·0.

Having performed his multiplications he gives London a bonus of 10%, other towns 2% and villages 1%. Lastly he estimates homeless people to number 80,000. The final result to the nearest round number is 5½ millions.

How King obtained his multiplier is not clear. In addition to the Hearth Office data he says he used 'the assessments on marriages, births, and burials, parish registers and other public accounts' and that from these he deduced the multipliers, but this is rather vague. He also classified the population by sex, civil state and age (under 1, under 5, under 10, under 16, above 16, above 21, above 25, above 60). How he reached these figures is not explained.

But nothing succeeds like success. As we shall see, his estimate of the total population is probably very near the truth and Prof. Westergaard has remarked that, judging from Swedish observations of a few years later, King's age distribution is quite reasonable.

As a statistical prophet King was no more successful than his contemporaries (and successors). He believed that down to his time the population of England had doubled in 435 years, that the next doubling would require from 1200 to 1300 years and that in A.D. 3500–3600 the population would reach 22 millions of souls, in case, as he cautiously adds 'the world should last so long'. His estimates as a matter of arithmetical curiosity are excellently fitted by a logistic with an upper asymptote of fifteen millions and would give the present population as about eight millions.

Modern statisticians, such as Farr and Brownlee, have confirmed King's estimate of the population at the end of the seventeenth century in the following

---

* Prof. E. C. K. Gonner (*J.R. Statist. Soc.* **76** (1912–13), 261–97), in an interesting paper which I have largely used in writing this chapter, remarks that the 'houses' of the Hearth Office must have been really families or separate occupations as King indeed realized, and thinks that King fell into some confusion in attempting to replace families by houses. Gonner argued that the best way was to proceed on the basis that the Hearth Office unit of a family should be retained and be corrected for empty houses, blacksmiths' shops, etc. on the basis of 1801 census returns and the multiplier used should be persons per family of 1801. The result is to give a figure about a quarter of a million larger than King's. The method described in the text also leads to the conclusion that King somewhat understated the population.

way. After 1801 the population was known by actual counting and for the first forty years of the nineteenth century baptisms and burials were still the only data of births and deaths. If one started from, say, the enumeration of 1831 and worked back to the population of 1821 by adding the numbers of burials and subtracting the number of baptisms then, if these really measured deaths and births, the result ought to agree with the census enumeration, provided immigration and emigration balanced. But the burials and baptisms understated deaths and births. One might adjust the figures by multipliers to bring the result into agreement with the census and then test against another backward run of ten years. Brownlee found that if the number of burials were multiplied by 1·2 and the number of baptisms by 1·243, the agreement was good.

This may seem a highly conjectural method, but it certainly gives quite good results. The difference between births and deaths estimated in this way for the decennium 1801–10, I find to be about 12·4 per 1000 living. If one multiplies the enumerated population of 1801 by $(1·0124)^{10}$ we reach 10·1 millions, not a bad approximation to 10·2 millions actually counted. Assuming that before 1801 burials and baptisms had the same relation to deaths and births as between 1801 and 1841, we can work backwards to the beginning of the eighteenth century with the result that the population then was about 5·8 millions, not much more than King's estimate. In view of the following discussion it will be useful to consider the probable state of the population (as determined by these methods) in the eighteenth century. In the first sixty years of the century it grew very slowly, was about 6·1 millions in 1751 and 6·5 millions in 1761. It then began to increase faster, was 7·5 in 1781, 8·2 by 1791 and 9·2 at the census of 1801 (8·9 as enumerated, but an estimate of a deficit of 1/30th was made).

From Gregory King's time to the census of 1801 we have a series of more or less intelligent guesses.

These are well described in Prof. Gonner's paper.* Two schools of thought did battle in the eighteenth century; the pessimists who held that the population was decreasing and the country going steadily to the dogs, and the optimists who believed just the contrary. Both used the same weapons. The heavy artillery was a return of houses for taxation purposes increased conjecturally by a figure for houses which escaped taxation, the sum multiplied by a conjectural average of persons per house. As light artillery one had the yield of taxes on commodities and the returns of baptisms and burials.

A pessimist put the number of untaxed houses low and the multiplier low, and an optimist raised both.

The first controversy which took place in 1754 in the proceedings of the Royal Society did not attract much notice. Brackenridge (mildly pessimistic) pointed out that the number of houses assessed to house tax had decreased between 1710 and 1754 from 729,048 to 690,000, which suggested a decrease of population (by a previous conjectural calculation based on burials and baptisms, he had

* *J.R. Statist. Soc.* **76** (1912–13), 261–96.

reckoned a small increase, which was probably correct). Much turned on the number of houses which did not pay tax (either because the occupant was in receipt of alms, did not, owing to poverty, contribute to the church or poor rate, or through mere default). Brackenridge put the number at 200,000. His critic, Forster, argued that Brackenridge under-stated the number of untaxed houses, adducing a sample of nine country parishes with 588 houses of which only 177 were taxed and a market town with 229 taxed houses out of 448. Using these figures as a basis for conjecture Forster raises Brackenridge's 890,000 to 1,427,110. From this (with a multiplier of 6 for town houses and 5 for country houses) he reaches a population of seven and a half millions—probably a considerable over-estimate.

The next controversy was a quarter of a century later (in a period when the population was certainly increasing) and its originator was Dr Richard Price (1723–91), who has attained a posthumous celebrity reminiscent of the man whose title to distinction was that he had once been kicked by George IV. Most readers know him as the preacher of a sermon which was the text of Burke's *Reflections*, most students of economic history know him as the inventor of that theory of the virtue of a Sinking Fund which has been likened to the economic system of a community which prospered by taking in one another's washing; most vital statisticians remember him as the computor of the Northampton Life Table which gave a seriously incorrect picture of prevailing mortality and in-directly cost the country a large sum of money. Finally, in the controversy about to be described, Price was pertinaciously in the wrong on all the main issues.

The apparent inference from all this is that Price was either a fool or a knave. West's portrait of the Rev. Richard Price, which hangs (or did hång) in the Board Room of the Equitable Assurance Society, gives no support to the hypothesis that Price was a fool; his life would be a promising field of research for a young historian with a competent knowledge of economics. His importance in statistical history is not great enough to justify me in a critical study (even if I had the necessary training in finance and economics). My guess is that Price was an able, self-confident, original-minded man, who knew a good deal about many things and had no exact knowledge of anything. He had 'a way' with him, he could *interest* people. In fact he had some of the qualities of Petty. It is easy enough to make jokes about his notion of the mysterious power of money to increase at compound interest and it is possible that William Pitt the younger (who was only a boy when he adopted Price's theory) was not a good economic reasoner. Still, even 150 years ago, there were bankers and Treasury officials, and it is possible that both they (and Price) were not so much bad theoretical reasoners as shrewd opportunists, that they were deliberately blind to the speciousness of an attractive defence of a desirable financial expedient. I have myself sometimes wondered whether, in the eighteenth century, an Assurance Society would have minded very much if a Life Table had erred on the pessimistic side.

Price did not enter on the population question with an unbiased mind. He was a keen politician and he believed that the policy of the government was bad for the country; he also believed that the wealth of a country was its people. Hence he believed that the population was declining and nothing shook that belief. Had he survived another ten years, until the first census, he would probably have disputed the accuracy of the returns.

Price began with the figures of houses in 1690, which he cited from Davenant (they were really due to King, who communicated them to Davenant), making the total 1,319,000. He then gave the figures of assessed, chargeable and cottages (cottages being houses too small to be taxed) as 678,915, 25,628 and 276,149, making a total of 980,692 in 1761. In 1777 they were 682,077, 19,396 and 251,261, a total of 952,734. On this basis he concluded that the population had declined by about one and a half millions and was actually less than five millions.

Howlett and Wales, Price's chief opponents, impugned every step in the reasoning. First, they pointed out that in the estimate for 1690 there was almost certainly a confusion between families and houses. Then they argued that many householders evaded duty (for instance by the simple plan of blocking up windows (the prayer 'Lighten our darkness, we beseech thee, Oh Pitt' is still remembered) and showed by direct enumeration in certain parishes that the returns were inaccurate. Finally, they gave reason to think that Price's multiplier was too small. On each of these points they were probably right. Indeed Price was obliged to admit the validity of some of their criticisms. But he declined to budge; sometimes he took *ad captandum* advantage of arithmetical slips by his adversaries, sometimes he declined to admit that their samples were representative, sometimes he tried to ignore the effect of corrections which he was forced to make.

These were the principal arguments. Both parties used the data of burials and baptisms as subsidiary arguments. Price seems only to have used the London Bills, which rather let him down; because although they seemed to help for some part of the century, he admits that by 1773 London was increasing and, very characteristically, uses this as in his favour: 'But it appears that, in truth, this is an event more to be dreaded than desired. The more London increases, the more the rest of the country must be deserted.' Price's adversaries went farther afield and counted burials and christenings in 162 parishes in all parts of England for two quinquennia, one beginning in 1758, the other in 1773. Baptisms increased from 47,638 to 59,567, burials from 49,553 to 53,030.

But neither party put much weight upon what we should now consider primary evidence; rightly, because of its incompleteness.

But these data were not wholly neglected by medical writers as we shall see in later sections. One may fairly say on the evidence here summarized that the eighteenth-century political arithmeticians of England made no advance whatever upon the position reached by Graunt, Petty and King. They were second-rate imitators of men of genius.

VI. SOME ENGLISH MEDICAL STATISTICIANS IN THE EIGHTEENTH CENTURY

AFTER Petty more than fifty years passed before another Fellow of the College of Physicians took an interest in statistics, and he, if less eminent in political arithmetic, was much more eminent in the art of medicine; he was the elder Heberden. Heberden published no statistical work over his name, but there seems no reason to doubt the accuracy of his son's statement that the quarto volume containing a collection of the yearly Bills of Mortality in London from 1657 to 1758 and various essays was financed by Dr William Heberden and that he wrote the preface. This preface, an essay of 15 pages which ends rather abruptly, could hardly have been written by a layman. The following passage illustrates my remark:

The deaths imputed to the measles are very remarkably different in different years; and yet it is possible that this disease is not in reality so very irregularly epidemical or fatal, as by the bills it appears to be. The scarlet fever and malignant sore throat often occasion such appearances upon the skin, as may easily be mistaken for the measles by better judges than the mothers and nurses, who thinking themselves able to distinguish this distemper, and equal to the management of it, often call in no other assistance. This mistake is well known to have been sometimes made within these few years, during which the scarlet fever and malignant sore throat have been so common. It may perhaps have happened in every year, in which an extraordinary number of deaths are charged to the measles: and consequently those two formidable distempers, (if they are two distinct distempers, and not one and the same) being disguised under the name of the measles, may have been older, and more general than is usually imagined.

The writer's observations upon the disappearance of plague have also something of a professional air—the fact that they are decidedly confused is no argument to the contrary. Sydenham taught (*Obs. Med.* **2**, 2) that plague depended upon (*a*) a special disposition of the atmosphere, (*b*) the transmission of an infecting matter, and held (*a*) to be primary, i.e. that without the atmospheric constitution there would be no epidemic. Heberden thinks the decline of the plague was due to the rebuilding of the city and—'probably the most effective'—the great quantity of water from the Thames and the New River, 'which, for the last century, has washed the houses so plentifully, and afterwards running down into the kennels and common sewers, constantly hinders, or weakens the tendency to putrefaction'. Heberden, unlike Sydenham, who believed the secret of the atmospheric constitution beyond the wit of man, seems to have attributed it to 'putrefaction', but, like Sydenham, attributed more importance to the atmospheric than the infective factor.

For the rest, Heberden continued Graunt's criticism of the material. In particular he gives good reason for thinking that beyond the omission of dissenters' christenings and burials, an important error arises from a balance of outward burials, that more coffins are taken out of London to be buried than are brought in. From an enumeration in Westminster he concludes that the deaths within the Bills are 20 % too few. He comments on an apparent increase in certain forms of death, such as apoplexies, lethargies and palsies. 'The practice of drinking spirituous liquors must, probably, answer for some part of this: and it might be of public use, if some attention were paid to the finding out of the other causes.' Rather optimistically, he thinks abundant amends might be made for these increases by the control of smallpox through inoculation. Upon this he makes a comment which has a very modern ring. 'For while inoculation prevails only among a part of any number of people, who all have an intercourse with one another, it may occasion as many deaths by spreading the distemper in, as it is called, the natural way, as it prevents among those, on whom it is practised.'

The volume contains a reprint of Graunt's work, of one of Petty's papers, and a new essay by Corbyn Morris. This essay, which shows signs of improving statistical technique, is not of medical interest except in its collection of deaths in age groups—an operation rendered possible by the introduction, in 1727, of an age classification of all deaths. Twelve age groups were given. In Heberden's preface the importance of classifying by cause of death and age is emphasized.

From this material a life table was calculated by a fellow of the Royal Society named Postlethwaite (at the request of Heberden). This table, based upon deaths alone, is, for reasons already stated, of little value.

I doubt whether even the relative mortalities are correctly shown. The age distribution of the Bills (after 1726) for deaths was: under 2, 2–5, 5–10 and thence forward by decennia. Consequently one must distribute the deaths into single years of life upon some principle of interpolation. Neither J.P. (Postlethwaite) nor J.S. (Smart)—who made a life table for the first ten of the thirty years—states the principle on which he worked. But J.P. assigns 250 of the 363 deaths at ages under 2 to the first year of life and J.S. 290 of the 386 he had to manipulate, respectively 68·9 and 75·1 % of the total mortality under 2. Both ratios are much less than given by Halley's table, 83·3 %, which itself agrees admirably with the latest English population table (E.L. No. 10, Males) 83·5 %. If we applied the 83 % ratio it would raise the rate of infant mortality to 301 per 1000. Taking the figures simply as they stand, the survivors to age 6 years are fewer than Graunt estimated—54 % not 64 % survive.

Although, as has been said, the arithmetical values are very suspect, the indication they give may be towards the truth. Creighton gave good reasons for concluding that London after the extinction of the Plague was less, not more, healthy. These reflexions are not without importance for they help to explain a certain fatalism, a scepticism as to the possibility of reducing the death-rate, which is noticeable in both statistical and medical literature for some time to come.

The next writer to be noticed is Thomas Short. Of this industrious investigator even Sir Norman Moore could obtain few personal particulars. He may have been born in 1690 and he died in 1772. He practised in Sheffield and was a Doctor of Medicine of a Scottish university but not a licentiate of the College. His principal works, *A General Chronological History of the Air, Weather, Seasons, Meteors, etc.*, published in 1749, and *New Observations, Natural, Moral, Civil, Political and Medical on City, Town and Country Bills of Mortality*, published in 1750, are differently assessed by the greatest historian of British medicine. Creighton pronounces the former to be rubbish but gives Short a not very hard pat on the back for the latter. 'That so much statistical or arithmetical zeal and exhaustiveness (in the work of 1750) should go with so total a deficiency of the critical and historical sense (in the work of 1749) is noteworthy, and perhaps not unparalleled in modern times' (Creighton, *Hist. of Epidem. in Britain*, 1, 405). Creighton's not very wide intellectual charity did not embrace statisticians.

It must be admitted that Short is decidedly *not* a writer to commend himself to an orderly minded, careful scholar from Aberdeen. Had he lived a century later we might have supposed that his literary model was Mrs Nickleby—he just runs on and on. A table (which must have been most troublesome to compile) of monthly christenings and weddings in various towns (in three extending over more than 150 years) leads him from arithmetical comparisons of the months most apt for procreation to a vigorous denunciation of luxury, of polygamy, of taxing common necessities, of the sale of army commissions, of novel reading, boarding schools and much else. But, although few if any would be able to read Short straight through without a rest, a good many less entertaining books might be included in a bed-side book case.

There is scarcely anything within the range of human interests upon which Dr Short has not something to say. On the whole he took a gloomy view of modern life in general and of his faculty in particular, and remarked that the 'improvements in surgery in general, have far out-stripped those in physick'. Surgeons he found to have generally less learning than physicians, but compensated for this by a closer application to the study of their own profession 'without jumbling the finite mind, and mixing studies of a different nature from their own, as of the dramatists, poets, classics, architecture, politics, history critics, logics, etc. They are also less liable to theories and false reasonings, have not that contempt of the ancients, nor of observations built on practice, improved and directed by the understanding, and raised to the pitch of truth by a long enquiry into the effects of diseases and medicines.'

Short began his book with a clear plan—long before he had finished it the plan became an inextricable confusion. He argued that a statistical measure of health could not be obtained from the data of towns in general and the capital in particular, partly owing to the inaccuracy of the data, partly owing to the fact that towns attracted newcomers and were not maintained by the balance of births and deaths within the community. So he collected material from country parishes (he also obtained data from towns but the country parishes were his prime object of study). His first set of data was a collection of transcripts of the registers of eighty-three parishes. About 60% of these parishes were from Yorkshire (mainly in the neighbourhood of Sheffield) and Derbyshire, but some from as far afield as Devonshire. He set them out in two periods, the first ending before the Restoration, the second coming down to the third decade of the eighteenth century. He had another set of eighty-three parishes for which the data covered only the second period. He classified his parishes in accordance with the nature of soil, altitude, exposure, whether wooded or bare, wet or dry. Sometimes his data covered more than a century, rarely less than 20 years. He gives the total number of baptisms, of burials (sexes distinguished) and marriages and works out the various ratios, the ratio of baptisms to burials being his chief tool.

From these data he draws a great many conclusions; for instance, respecting the salubrity or insalubrity of different soils and exposures. Most of these conclusions, it may be remarked, are now part of the common stock of lay and, perhaps, professional belief. But whether Short's data were adequate to sustain the conclusions is another question.

We may begin by taking purely arithmetical points into consideration, viz. whether, *assuming* that the parishes or groups of parishes were fairly comparable and *assuming* that the ratio of baptisms to burials is a fair measure of healthiness, Short had large enough figures for his purpose. For instance, two of his conclusions were that dry open sites of moderate elevation were healthier than a clay soil. I picked out of his list nine parishes of the former and five of the latter class. In his first (pre-Restoration) period, the parishes on dry, open sites had registered 4349 baptisms and 2644 burials, a ratio of 1·64. The five parishes on clay had 2875 baptisms and 1920 burials, a ratio of 1·497. So, as he said, the dry open sites give a higher ratio. But what is the order of magnitude of the error of sampling? We may safely hold that the standard error of the number of baptisms or burials is of the order of the square root of the observed number, or the ratio of standard error to number is of order $1/n^{\frac{1}{2}}$. From this we infer that the standard error of the ratio n_1/n_2 is given by n_1/n_2 times $(1/n_1 + 1/n_2 - 2r_{n_1 n_2} . 1/(n_1 n_2)^{\frac{1}{2}})^{\frac{1}{2}}$. Clearly, the correlation between numerator and denominator must be large, so that the second factor lies between $(1/n_1 + 1/n_2)^{\frac{1}{2}}$ and $(1/n_1^{\frac{1}{2}} - 1/n_2^{\frac{1}{2}})$ and will be much nearer the second value. In a sample of 1000 Registration Districts I studied many years ago, the correlation of births and deaths was 0·73%, in our particular case the standard error of the difference between the two ratios will be likely to be not much more than 20% of its value.

From the purely arithmetical angle, I should conclude that Short was justified in holding that his ratios did really differ significantly, as we say, from site to site. But is it fair to assume that (1) the ratio of baptisms to burials is a good index of healthiness, (2) that the comparisons are in *pari materia*? These are much more difficult questions.

So far as concerns modern experience, it is clear that the ratio of births to deaths does not give a useful index of the rate of mortality. I made an experiment on Short's lines. I took out a sample of fifty Registration Districts for the decennium 1901–10, chosen in the following way. (1) No districts with more than 10,000 births or fewer than 1000 deaths were taken. (2) Those with many institutional deaths were excluded. For each the ratio of births to deaths was calculated and the following table formed:*

Ratio of births to deaths	No. of districts	Mean of standardized death-rates
2·0–	4	10·36
1·9–	6	10·88
1·8–	7	11·04
1·7–	6	11·60
1·6–	15	11·15
1·5–	7	10·72
1·4–	4	11·48
1·3–	1	13·01

It is true that the district with highest ratio has the lowest death-rate and the district with lowest ratio the highest death-rate, but in detail there is but little correspondence. Testing the same districts on the data of 30 years earlier, 1871–80, the same result appears. It would be very rash to conclude that because a district has a ratio of births to deaths above the average its standardized death-rate is below the average.

There are many reasons why a ratio of births to deaths may be a bad measure and Short knew this; for instance, the deaths might be increased by immigrants or decreased by emigrants. He was a true Englishman of Whig principles, and in speaking of *foreign* registers, remarks that 'where the births vastly exceed the burials, the country is either very healthy, or it is under an arbitrary government or both'. If the former, the marriages will bear a high proportion to the baptisms, few will die in infancy. If the latter, 'tho' more males are born, yet the funerals of females far exceed them; there is little industry amongst

* The districts selected were: Hambledon, Malling, Faversham, Romney Marsh, Uckfield, New Forest, Romsey, Hartley Wintry, Royston, Winslow, Witney, Oundle, St Ives, Caxton, Whittlesea, Lexden, Risbridge, Mildenhall, Bosmere, Plomesgate, Flegg, Cricklade, Melksham, Amesbury, Sturminster, Kingsbridge, Stratton, St Columb, Langport, Dursley, Ledbury, Wem, Mastley, Meriden, Shipston on Stour, Lutterworth, Spilsby, Hayfield, Garstang, Settle, Pateley Bridge, Gt Ouseburn, Saddleworth, Thorne, Pocklington, Skirlaugh, Easingwold, Bedale, Weardale, Brampton.

the people, because they want property; useless standing armies are kept up in time of peace, for the grandeur of the tyrant, maintaining his tyranny and the oppression of his people'.

Quite logically he argues that if the burials greatly exceed the baptisms, either the situation is unhealthy or the government is limited (i.e. on English lines). One diagnoses the former when epidemics are frequent and the proportion of deaths in youth and childhood large; 'the latter is known from the great resort of strangers, labourers, artificers, merchants, etc., increase of business, trade and riches; or there is a large body of people mixed with the society, of different manners and principles, whose baptisms are not registered with the rest'.

Short was, then, aware of the fallacies possible, but he held that in country parishes they were not important.

I am not confident that he was wrong so far as concerns his first period data; country villages from the middle of the sixteenth century to the middle of the seventeenth century. But when we come to the next 80 years, when England was beginning to be an industrial country, the assumptions are more hazardous, and the almost invariably pessimistic conclusions he draws (it is a little odd that the population pessimists did not make more use of Short) may well be fallacious. The cause of change for the worse was, in the first place, the deluge of profaneness which came with the Restoration, in the next place the increase of 'Luxury, pride, intemperance and debauchery' associated with the growth of industry and wealth, so fortunately associated with the 'happy Revolution' and stabilized by the 'seasonable Accession of the present Royal Family'. But Short charges this intemperance and debauchery particularly upon the towns, and it does seem a little unreasonable to suppose that even the happy Revolution or the Hanoverian accession much increased the opportunities of villagers to fall into the sins of luxury and pride.

Short next considers the succession of unhealthy years in villages and towns. He nowhere states what his criterion of a sickly year was. The arm-chair statistician might suppose that he would take a ratio of baptisms to burials which fell below some assigned percentage of the average; but, in default of any specific statement, I should guess that Short called a year sickly when the burials exceeded the baptisms; since his totals show always an excess of baptisms over burials, this would seem a simple rule. But he may have been more subtle. He remarks: 'It may be a sickly or mortal year in a town or country parish and yet the christenings may exceed the buryings considerably, either because it happens to be a very fruitful year in that place (as often tho' not generally happens) or the year may be very sickly in that parish, if compared with other years, and yet healthy if compared with other places in much worse situations and air.' This suggests that a sudden rise in the number of burials would be his criterion, and I have found half a dozen cases in his table (of nearly 400 instances,

viz. country registers and market-town registers, examined from 1541 to 1741)
when the burials for sickly years did not exceed the christenings.

It is a pity Short was not more explicit; his work in this field was original
and suggestive. He finds that in the country parishes the frequency of unhealthy
years is never more than twice in 5 or 6 and often as rarely as once in 6 or 8
years, 'which is indeed as long, if not a longer interval, than commonly happens
between one visitation of smallpox and measles and another, exclusive of all
other diseases'. 'When sickly years return oftenest there is a less disproportion
between christenings and burials than when they come seldomest.' Healthy places
have 'their frequent eruptive and inflammatory diseases', unhealthy places 'their
slow intermittents, remittents, putrid and erratic fevers'. 'It is true, some rare
times the former places are visited with the latter diseases, but rarely except
they are epidemics; nor are they of a great spread, duration or execution. The
latter's places have also the former's diseases, but (eruptive fevers excepted)
more mildly and rarely; for each country or situation is more liable to some
diseases than others, and by traffic and commerce endemics became epidemics,
as far as air and climate will allow.' Short passes to a general survey of epidemiological history which is not, I think, without value, but has, of course, long
been superseded by Creighton's classical study.

The passages upon which I have commented are all from the first quarter of
Short's treatise and typify, I think, his most valuable contributions to our
subject. As his book proceeds, not only does his habit of improving the occasion
grow upon him but, in commenting and performing arithmetical operations upon
the London Bills, he does not show to great advantage. But anybody who will
trouble to dip into the book is likely to make a friend. Creighton said of him
that 'his abstract results or conclusions are colourless and unimpressive, as
statistical results are apt to be for the average concrete mind'. This seems to me
rather misleading. I dare say nobody ever burst into tears over or was thrown
into paroxysms of mirth by a statistical table—even a table compiled by the
Army Medical Department. It is quite likely that several of Short's inferences
were wrong. But he *did* paint a vivid picture of the changing conditions of life
as he saw it. 'Colourless' is about the last adjective I should apply to his book.
Had it been studied with more attention, had he been a leading London
physician instead of an obscure country practitioner, medical statistics in
England would have progressed faster.

VII. SOME REPRESENTATIVE CONTINENTAL DEMOGRAPHERS
OF THE EIGHTEENTH CENTURY

My object is to sketch the history of distinctively medical statistics in our
own country; I have neither the knowledge nor, perhaps, the desire to cover a
wider field; but it would be too insular entirely to neglect continental research
contemporaneous with that described in the preceding section. I propose to

discuss the work of some foreign writers which is relevant to that of the British authors mentioned in the preceding section. The most eminent contemporaries of Short were Deparcieux, Wargentin, Struyck, Kerseboom and Süssmilch, and of these Deparcieux, Struyck and Süssmilch are, I think, the most interesting, a Frenchman, a Hollander and a German. None of them was a physician. Deparcieux and Struyck were competent mathematicians. Struyck wrote on the general theory of probability, Süssmilch had no more mathematics than Graunt; but, of the three, Süssmilch is better known to posterity because he is frequently cited in books which circulate outside professional statistical circles. Deparcieux (1703–68) is the least voluminous and most attractive of the three. He published in 1746 a quarto of 132 pages (with tables) entitled *Essai sur les Probabilités de la Durée de la Vie humaine*, to which he added, 14 years later, a short appendix, and his book is a model of clear writing.

Deparcieux was fully alive to the dangers of basing a life table upon data of mortality alone, and was the first writer to construct what we should regard now (subject to a few reservations) as correct tables. Of course, like his contemporaries, he could not make bricks without straw, and no more than they could provide a general population life table. He had to use data which were not random samples of human experience and is careful to point this out. His new material was drawn from two sources, the data of tontines and the mortality experience of religious orders.

A tontine (the name is derived from that of the inventor Lorenzo Tonti, a Neapolitan banker) was a system of selling annuities on the following plan. The participants are formed into age classes, each entrant pays a capital sum and receives an annuity; as the annuitants die out the amount payable to the survivors is increased and the last survivor will enjoy an income equal to that distributed originally over all members of the age class. This was the general plan of a simple tontine (*The Wrong Box* will have made us familiar with a different application); there were various modifications, but in all an exact record of deaths at ages was essential.

Deparcieux used the data of tontines established in 1689 and 1696. He had to face many difficulties. In the first place, the tontines had a series of classes, one for those entrants under the age of 5, the next for lives from 5 to 10, and so on. What is the mean age of the members of each class? There would, as Deparcieux points out, be a bias in the first class (that of children under 5) in favour of ages beyond the mean, because parents needed no statistics to convince them that the rate of mortality in the first and second years of life is higher than in the third and fourth or fifth. In the later classes, on the other hand, the bias would be in favour of entering at an age below the mean of the class limits. He makes a rather modest allowance for these factors by taking the age at entrance in the first class as 3 years, i.e. half a year more than the mean of the class limits, and in the next (and subsequent classes) as half a year less than the mean. The next difficulty is that his observations end in 1742, consequently rates of mortality at ages are derived from persons whose dates of birth are widely separated. Thus no members of the first class of the 1689 tontine can have been exposed to the risk of dying at ages beyond 57 (actually of 202 entrants, 105 were still living at the close of the observations). So a table obtained by welding these observations ignores any secular trend of mortality. It also ignores what, in modern assurance practice, is an important factor, viz. selection. A life aged *n* years is less likely to end within the year of entrance than a life of the same age entered 10 years earlier. In ordinary practice there are two reasons, self-selection and medical examination. In annuitant experience only the former is involved, but this is not the *less* important of the two.

In the discussion of this subject which will be found in Elderton and Oakley's *The Mortality of Annuitants* 1900–1920 (published on behalf of the Institute of Actuaries in 1924), the conclusion is reached that when *contemporaneous* lives are in question, this selection only operates seriously on the first year of annuitant life; for that year the rate of mortality is about 63 % of that suffered by annuitants of the same age who had purchased annuities 5 years earlier (what is called ultimate mortality). If then there were no secular improvement of mortality rates—as there has been over the last 60 years—and if there were no secular change in the social or economic class of annuitants, while we should expect a lighter mortality upon recent entrants, if, as in Deparcieux's data, we are only given survivors at quinquennial intervals, we should not expect large differences. Actually one can test a particular age group, viz. 45–50 on numerically extensive material. The 1689 tontine provides ten and the 1696 tontine nine groups of persons of this age the survivors of which 5 years later are recorded. It will be seen from Table 1 that the 634 'new' entrants in the 45–50 tontine class of 1689 suffered rather heavier mortality than the 118 survivors to that age from the youngest class. This, however, is merely picking out a single pair. The correct test is to treat the data together and inquire whether the hypothesis that the whole set of deaths and survivorships might have arisen by sampling a population for which the chance of living 5 years was simply the ratio of total survivors to total exposed, viz. $5009/5394 = 0.9286$. Applying the appropriate test, viz. that known as the χ^2 test (with 18 degrees of freedom), one reaches $P = 0.0346$. This is not a very improbable freak of chance. Compared with modern annuitants, these tontiniers of 200 years ago had a rate of mortality some 40 % greater than the annuitants of 1900–20 between the ages of 47 and 52.

Finally, one has the class of society from which annuitants are drawn. Deparcieux was of opinion that annuitants were mainly drawn (op. cit. p. 62) from the middle class of society 'ce sont les bons Bourgeois qui tiennent un honnête milieu entre toutes ces extremités, qui se font des Rentes viagères; et ce sont ceux-là qui deviennent ordinairement vieux'. Hence he judged that the rate of mortality suffered would be less than that of the general population.

Table 1. *Deparcieux's observations*

Tontine class	Exposed to risk at age 47	Survivors to age 52		Deaths	
		Observed	Expected	Observed	Expected
(1689 tontine)					
− 5	118	109	110	9	8
−10	181	173	168	8	13
−15	211	192	196	19	15
−20	216	196	201	20	15
−25	201	189	187	12	14
−30	263	249	244	14	19
−35	526	479	488	47	38
−40	472	440	438	32	34
−45	770	723	715	47	55
−50	634	575	589	59	45
(1696 tontine)					
5–10	134	130	124	4	10
−15	131	118	122	13	9
−20	108	103	100	5	8
−25	102	92	95	10	7
−30	147	135	137	12	10
−35	211	204	196	7	15
−40	220	200	204	20	16
−45	444	415	412	29	32
−50	305	287	283	18	22
	5394	5009		385	

The next part of his investigation related to the mortality experience of members of monastic orders. These he utilized with the same good sense and care.

In Table 2 are his l_x values, to which I have added those for English Life Table No. 9 Males (general mortality of 1930–2). The reason for putting l_{20} equal to 814 is simply that in his table for tontines where the starting point is age 3, his survivors to age 20 from an initial 1000 were 814.

The column headed Benedictines (*a*) is a methodologically correct table, viz. based on entrants followed until death, Benedictines (*b*) assumes a stationary population and is not therefore so exact although it utilizes more data. Actually both tables give virtually the same results. It will be seen that to age 50 all the tables agree well; after age 50 the monks fare worse than the members of tontines and worse than the nuns. All have much worse mortality than the unselected general population of England and Wales 200 years later. Deparcieux attributes to selection the equality of tontine and monastic mortalities at younger ages and to the privations and austerities of the religious life a higher mortality at later ages.

In an investigation made by Dr S. Monckton Copeman and myself some years ago (*Report on Public Health and Medical Subjects*, no. 36, H.M.S.O. 1926) into the alleged low mortality from cancer of members of certain religious orders, we had occasion to study the general mortality experience. The result was that the mortality at ages over 25 of monks was rather more favourable than that of

Table 2. *Deparcieux's observations*

| Age | Tontines | Survivors from age 20 | | Nuns | E.L. No. 9 Males |
		Bene-dictines (a)	Bene-dictines (b)		
20	814	814	814	814	814
30	734	756	749	751	788
40	657	675	681	676	755
50	581	575	583	587	698
60	463	423	432	462	594
70	310	236	235	286	405
80	118	55	51	103	151

annuitants, that of nuns less favourable. The data were, however, scanty (monks 65 observed against 79·4 expected deaths; nuns 152 observed against 124·7 expected deaths).

Deparcieux has a few remarks on general medical-statistical questions (for instance, he urges strongly the importance of mothers nursing their infants), but nothing of much significance.

The statistical writings of Nicholas Struyck (1687–1769) are more voluminous than those of Deparcieux* and cover a wider field. Struyck was the son of an Amsterdam burgher and is said to have been in relatively easy circumstances. He enjoyed a considerable reputation as a writer on mathematical, statistical, geographical and astronomical subjects and was admitted a fellow of the Royal Society of London in 1749.

Struyck was evidently a competent mathematician and also an industrious field worker who carried out or inspired in the Netherlands many town and village enumerations of population and vital statistical records. Like Deparcieux, he constructed life tables from annuitants' data and he certainly understood the correct arithmetical procedure. His data were, however, much fewer and he does not give sufficient details of his methods of interpolation and approximation to central ages for it to be possible to say precisely how he reached the life tables for males and females printed on p. 231 of his book. The original data

* They were collected and published in French translation at the instance of the Netherlands Assurance Society in 1912: *Les Œuvres de Nicolas Struyck, qui rapportent au calcul des chances*, etc., traduites du Hollandais par J. A. Vollgraff, Amsterdam, 1912, pp. 430.

were 794 males and 876 females (annuitants) observed for various periods and classified in quinquennial age groups. One has the impression that, although Struyck was a mathematician, he was not very sensitive to the dangers of basing conclusions upon small absolute numbers, and in his discussion of the vital statistics of London (op. cit. pp. 348–51) he has hardly given enough weight to the disturbing influence of migration and is perilously near the fallacy of a stationary population.

From the point of view of the medical statistician, Struyck is not a very suggestive writer. As demographer, we might rank him as technically superior to Short but medically less interesting. Like his contemporaries he can chase' phantom hares in a thoroughly entertaining way. His finest example is in a section on multiple births. After a sober statistical inquiry he concludes that a case of quintuplets might reasonably be expected to occur sometimes in populations of the sizes of those of France and Germany—'it would be a very rare but not an incredible event'.

The case of the countess of Hennenberg, alleged to have brought to birth 364 or 365 infants simultaneously, does, however, strike him as 'absolutely fantastic and contrary to nature', and he carefully examines the legend. The statement was that the prolific mother produced as many children as the days of the year, and that the boys were named John and the girls Elizabeth. As Struyck justly observes it would be silly to have 182 Johns and 182 Elizabeths, and by careful research he arrives at a simple rational solution. The lady performed her feat on 26 March 1266; at that period the year began with the Feast of the Annunciation which was 25 March. So the birthday was the *second* day of the year and probably the mother had twins, one christened John the other Elizabeth. *Simplex munditiis!*

The name of Johann Peter Süssmilch (1707–67) is far better known than those of Deparcieux and Struyck although it is doubtful whether his *book* is often read. The perusal of 1201 pages of text and 207 of tables (the contents of the third edition of Süssmilch's book, published in 1765) requires a powerful appetite. If Süssmilch's literary style has less complexity than that of successors who wrote after German had become a 'literary' language, it has not much charm and few of us love propaganda. Süssmilch is a pure propagandist; the title of his book is: 'Die göttliche Ordnung in den Veränderungen des menschlichen Geschlechts, aus der Geburt, dem Tode und der Fortpflanzung desselben *erwiesen*' (italics mine), von Johann Peter Süssmilch. He sets out to reveal the divine machinery for fulfilling the command: 'Be fruitful, and multiply, and replenish the earth, and subdue it.' The reason why his book has more interest for a statistician than, say, Warburton's *Divine Legation*, is that Süssmilch conceived the notion that vital statistics might be pressed into the service of orthodox Lutheran theology, and the diligence with which he pursued his arithmetical investigations gave his book importance. It was indeed the quarry from which Malthus obtained material when the interest aroused by the first edition of his famous *Essay* led him to expand what had been not much more than a Shavian paradox into a serious treatise.

As a demographer and statistician, Süssmilch was technically inferior to either Deparcieux or Struyck and, of course, far below Halley. He had none of Graunt's originality and made no methodological advance. But he was very industrious. He assembled not only a large collection of German data, similar to but wider than those of Short, but collected foreign material—including that of Graunt, King and Short—and his tables are of real value.

The general conclusions he reached—constancy of the sex ratio, greater mortality of towns, etc.—differ in no important respect from those of his predecessors or English contemporaries. His own life table (which gave an expectation of life at birth of 28·43 years) is constructed on the incorrect principles adopted by most of his contemporaries. He was, indeed, aware that to make a life table by summing the deaths at ages occurring in an increasing population was wrong and that the population he used was increasing, but he did not know how to do better—indeed, he had no material for doing better.

His contribution to purely medical statistics is small. He has a chapter on the statistics of causes of death and compares the distribution by causes in the London Bills 1728–57 with those for Berlin in the years 1745, 1750 and 1757. When allowance is made for differences of nomenclature and misprints, the proportional distributions by causes are not very different. He makes the sensible suggestion that if the Latin names of the diseases were given by the medical attendants in official returns international comparison would be facilitated. For the rest, his medical importance is slight. To criticize or make fun of his triumphant justification of the ways of God to man would be sorry trifling. Although a dull writer, he inspires a certain affection. He was a sincere, diligent man and in polemics more courteous than most. He may, perhaps, quite contrary to his intention, have had a rather depressing influence upon enthusiastic readers, in that he had no expectation of a great reduction of mortality rates and has often anticipated ideas which we usually attribute to Malthus. He perceived that at the current rate of growth the earth must eventually be overpopulated, but he argued that as the density of population increased the age of marriage would rise and consequently the fertility rate would decline. 'If, however, fertility remained the same, it would only be necessary for the rate of mortality to increase a little, so that, as in large towns, one in 25 died' (op. cit. 1, 267).

He devotes a whole chapter to what Malthus would call positive checks upon population and clearly does not expect these to be eliminated although, for the reason just quoted, he does not think plagues and wars essential conditions. One, perhaps only one, item of the vital statistical system gave the good man some qualms. His arithmetic leads him to conclude that in cities half those born are dead by the 20th year of life, and even in the virtuous country districts half are dead before the age of 25. 'What is the reason that God permits half to die before they can be of service to God and the world? All the labour and effort of birth and rearing seem to have been in vain' (op. cit. **2**, 312). In a worldly sense there is, he confesses, no explanation. One must think of earthly life as but a preparation for the hereafter.

The trend of this reasoning is not encouraging to the social or hygienic reformer. Perhaps Süssmilch did contribute a little to the view that not much could be done to reduce the general death-rate, that, at the best, town death-rates might be slightly improved. But I doubt whether he had much influence upon medical opinion in England. Statistics are not even now a favourite study of the medical profession; 200 years ago a voluminous German writer on vital statistics would have found very few readers in the College of Physicians.

VIII. METHODOLOGICAL ADVANCES

The writers who were the subject of the last sections all flourished in the first half of the eighteenth century and all have a claim to be reckoned as pioneers. Deparcieux and Struyck made definite contributions to the mathematical or arithmetical technique of life-table construction; Süssmilch and Short followed the path blazed by Graunt, but they explored a good deal of country, and Short, at least, had novel ideas as to the utilization of local records.

In the later years of the century various medical writers, for instance, Heysham, Haygarth and Percival, made effective use of local enumerations of population in their efforts to secure sanitary improvements. The public has no passion for statistics, still a death-rate *is* more telling than a mere enumeration of deaths. But none of these writers contributed anything new to statistical methodology, and simple arithmetic, not to speak of the labour of making unofficial counts of population, is not every man's hobby. Had the proposal for making an official census in the middle of the century been accepted, no doubt interest in political or medical arithmetic would have revived, but it did not pass the House of Lords. The only official data of large dimensions were still the London Bills. These were sometimes the subject of medical statistical comment. In 1800, the younger Heberden wrote a monograph the title of which suggested competition with Short or even Graunt. But it was not a successful venture and is only remembered now (if at all) because of a statistical 'howler' which the iconoclastic Charles Creighton exposed with a satisfaction not melancholy.* ·

A typical example of the attitude of the better class of physicians towards statistics at the end of the eighteenth century will be found in *Observations Medical and Political on the Small-Pox...and on the Mortality of Mankind at*

* *Vide supra*, p. 28.

every Age in City and Country..., by W. Black, M.D., the second edition of which appeared in 1781. Dr Black, a medical graduate of Leyden and a licentiate of the College, who survived to 1829, reprinted the life tables of his predecessors. He was alive to the importance of the statistical method and its neglect ('In the course of many years' attendance upon medical lectures, in different universities, I never once heard the bills of mortality mentioned', op. cit. p. 119) and held that 'the detached observations of physicians or other literary individuals, confined perhaps to a small town or parish: a meagre detail of village remarks (*sic*), afford in many instances a foundation too slight to erect upon them any general or permanent conclusions' (op. cit. p. 119). He accordingly devoted most of his attention to the London Bills, which he subjected to a severe but cogent criticism, and set out in detail a sensible plan for the compilation of data in London by salaried officials with medical knowledge, which, had it been adopted, would have antedated the establishment of effective registration in London by more than 50 years.

One might explain the stagnation of medical statistical research by saying that there was not enough straw for ordinary brick makers to be employed, and no medical man of sufficient ingenuity (or temerity) to find a substitute for straw emerged. If that eminent fellow and, for a very short space of time, president of the College James Jurin had lived in the second instead of the first half of the eighteenth century, it is possible that the history of medical statistics would have been different, because, some years after his death, two famous mathematicians tackled a problem in which Jurin had taken keen interest and, as he himself was an accomplished mathematician, their method would have given him intellectual pleasure.

Jurin was an enthusiastic supporter of the practice of smallpox inoculation and wished to provide an adequate statistical proof of its value. Monk provides an eulogistic, Creighton a depreciatory account of what Jurin did. A fuller account is given by Miss Karn (M. N. Karn, *Ann. Eugen.* 4 (1931), 279 et seq.).

That Jurin proved the fatality of inoculated smallpox to be very much less than that of the natural smallpox, even Creighton admitted. But that he did much more can hardly be claimed. Jurin virtually assumed that inoculated smallpox did confer an immunity, on the basis of others' testimony and the famous experiment on six criminals, or rather on the one criminal who after inoculation was deliberately exposed to natural infection (see Creighton, op. cit. p. 480). Whether Jurin deserves to be sneered at because he did not do what was impossible, or whether the assumptions he made were unreasonable, are questions I shall not discuss. The mathematicians added nothing to the biological discussion, the interest of their work is purely intellectual, viz. by showing how to make the most of imperfect material. The problem proposed by Daniel Bernoulli was this.

Let us assume that inoculation completely protects against dying from smallpox and that those who are thus saved from the smallpox are neither more nor less likely to die of other causes than persons who never take smallpox, then what would be the effect on general mortality of the total eradication of small-pox? Put more picturesquely, how many years would be added to the average span of human life if smallpox were extinct?

In modern times, questions like this have often been put and answered, because we know with fair accuracy the numbers living by sex and age and the numbers dying from different causes also by sex and age. In the famous Supplement to the 35*th Annual Report of the Registrar-General*, Farr dealt with several causes. His method was simple. He subtracted from the central death-rate at any age due to all causes of death the central death-rate due to the special cause, and deduced from the resultant series of modified death-rates the appropriate life table constants. These he compared with those of the general life table. He found in this way that if phthisis were eliminated the expectation of life at birth (males) would be increased from 39·7 to 43·96 years. The elimina-tion of the zymotic diseases would increase the mean lifetime to 46·77 years.

Farr was, of course, aware that the assumption, viz. if a particular cause of mortality was eliminated the death-rates from other diseases would not be affected, might not be justified—indeed, he had written with respect of Watt's lugubrious substitution theory, in accordance with which we gain little by eliminating one disease, its killing power will be taken by another. Farr's method is quite satisfactory as an arithmetical method but requires data not available in the eighteenth century. Bernoulli made two assumptions. The first that mortality rates from all causes were known (for his arithmetical calculations he used Halley's table although he did not quite correctly appreciate the meaning of Halley's phrase 'age current'), the second that the attack and fatality rates of smallpox were independent of age. He then reasoned thus:

Suppose there survive to age x by the life table P_x persons. Of these s, say, have not had smallpox; if $1/n$th of those who have not had smallpox were attacked within a year and $1/m$th of these die of smallpox, what is the value of s in terms of P_x, m and n? If dx is an element of time, $s\,dx/n$ will be attacked and $s\,dx/(mn)$ will die of smallpox within the element of time dx, and so there die from other diseases $-dP_x - s\,dx/(mn)$ because $-dP_x$ is the total mortality. But we are only interested in s, so the decrement through mortality $-dP_x - s\,dx/(mn)$ must be multiplied by s/P_x, and we reach the equation

$$-ds = \frac{s\,dx}{n} - \frac{s}{P_x}\left(dP_x + \frac{s\,dx}{mn}\right),$$

the solution of which is
$$s = \frac{mP_x}{(m-1)\,e^{x/n} + 1}.$$

So s is known. Now let z be the number who would have survived to age x had there been no smallpox. Reasoning as before

$$-dz = -\frac{z}{P_x}\left(dP_x + \frac{s\,dx}{mn}\right).$$

The integral of which is
$$z = \frac{P_x m\, e^{x/n}}{(m-1)\, e^{x/n} + 1}.$$

This is the solution. Bernoulli put $n = m = 8$ and concluded that the elimination of smallpox would, on these assumptions, add about 3 years to the mean life-time.

D'Alembert criticized Bernoulli's assumption that m and n were constant and replaced his equation by the formally simpler equation

$$dz = \frac{z}{P_x}\,dP_x + \frac{z}{P_x}\,du,$$

where du is the increment of mortality in time dx due to smallpox. The formal solution is
$$z = P_x \exp\left[\int_0^x \frac{du}{P_x}\right].$$

Isaac Todhunter commented sub-acidly on this: 'The result is not of practical use because the value of the integral is not known. D'Alembert gives several formulae which involve this or similar unfinished integrations' (*History of the Theory of Probability*, p. 268). Todhunter's comment is just so far as concerns the situation when Bernoulli and D'Alembert wrote. If, in addition to a table of general mortality, one has knowledge of the deaths at ages due to smallpox, then by means of the theorem known as the Euler-Maclaurin expansion, it *is* possible to evaluate the integral and reach a solution on D'Alembert's lines as Miss Karn (op. cit. pp. 303 et seq.) has shown. But if we do have this information, the much less laborious method of Farr is adequate.

But that does not mean that the attempt of Bernoulli and D'Alembert was futile, a mere display of mathematical fireworks. The situation in which they found themselves recurs time and again in the history of statistics, indeed of all branches of science. Often a practical man objects that a mathematician will write down equations in general terms which cannot be solved and are therefore, as the practical man urges, of no use to him. Sometimes the practical man is right, but not always; not even usually. Even when the equations cannot be solved, in the sense that certain 'constants' cannot be determined or certain integrals evaluated, methods of approximation, even inspired guesses, may lead to truth. Fifty years after Bernoulli and D'Alembert, E. E. Duvillard* published a monograph which, although seldom read, for it is scarce and 'practically' obsolete, has been rightly described by Farr as a classic of vital statistics. Duvillard set himself the same problem with the difference that vaccination was substituted for inoculation as the prophylactic, and this book, of nearly 200 quarto pages, may still be read with profit.

* *Analyse et tableaux de l'influence de la petite vérole sur la mortalité à chaque âge*, Paris, 1806.

Duvillard lived before the days of Cauchy and mathematical rigour; no doubt much of his work would hardly satisfy the standard of a modern pure mathematician. Perhaps on that account it can be read by the amateur with comparative ease, and one may take hints of how to tackle problems for the solution of which complete statistical data are still to seek. There is no proverb the vital or medical statistician should more often repeat than the saying that the best is often the enemy of the good. It is no doubt foolish to suppose, as, according to Isaac Todhunter, Condorcet did suppose, that truth could be extracted from any data, however imperfect, provided one used formulae garnished with a sufficient number of signs of integration. It is more foolish to neglect even rough approximations to unattainable solutions. But, so far as concerns our predecessors in the College, indeed in the medical profession as a whole, the seed scattered by the foreign mathematicians fell upon stony ground. Between Short and Farr, no British physician made a contribution to statistical knowledge of much importance. I have spoken of the younger Heberden's brochure. William Woolcombe of Plymouth, writing on the alleged increase of tuberculosis,* showed a better grasp of statistical method than the more famous physician.

The question Woolcombe examined was whether mortality from tuberculosis of the lungs were increasing. The statistical fact was that in well-kept registers he had examined the proportion of deaths assigned to consumption had certainly increased towards the end of the eighteenth century. Woolcombe was alive to the fact (often ignored by medical writers after his time) that the proportional mortality of a disease might increase although its absolute rate of mortality was stationary or even diminishing, and he tested his conclusions by a quite logical *ex absurdo* argument. Taking the assumption that at the beginning of the eighteenth century mortality was 1 in 36 and that the proportional mortality from phthisis was a third less than in 1801, he concluded that the general rate of mortality at the beginning of the nineteenth century must be as low as 1 in 54, unless the rate of mortality from phthisis had increased. But it was certain that in 1800 the general rate of mortality was higher than 1 in 54, at least 1 in 47. Reversing the process, viz. assuming the rate in 1801 to be known, the conclusion was reached that the rate of mortality at the beginning of the eighteenth century must have been 1 in 27 unless the rate of mortality from phthisis had increased. This Woolcombe thought improbably high. He may have been wrong, but his method was rational. That was the best piece of medical statistical reasoning I have found in English medical literature between Short and Farr.

In 1800 the taking of a census was authorized by the legislature and not a government department, but the Speaker of the House of Commons was charged with the responsibility. Naturally, Mr Speaker passed over the actual work to one of his subordinates, and fortunately that subordinate, John Rickman, whose

---

* *The Frequency and Fatality of Different Diseases, Particularly on the Progressive Increase of Consumption, with Observations on the Influence of the Seasons on Mortality.* 155 pp. London, 1808.

name is immortalized by the fact that he was a friend and correspondent of Charles Lamb, was really interested in statistics. In the report on the enumeration of 1801 comments are scanty, but they increased in subsequent volumes. Rickman was wholly responsible for the work down to the report of 1831 and, although he made no advance in statistical method, he did valuable work, particularly in calling attention to the high rate of mortality in the industrial north-west and in estimating past populations of the country. But Rickman was not professionally interested in medical questions, and before Farr no medical man utilized the new material effectively. As will be seen in the next section, the first English writer to publish a work under the title Medical Statistics was rather old fashioned in his treatment of the subject.

IX. THE END OF AN EPOCH

Almost at the end of the period I have chosen was published the first English book specifically devoted to Medical Statistics, *Elements of Medical Statistics*, by F. Bisset Hawkins, printed in 1829. It is a slender volume of 233 pages similar in format and size to the *Principles of Medical Statistics* published a little more than a century later, in 1937, by my friend and colleague Dr A. Bradford Hill.

Hawkins's book was an expansion of the Gulstonian Lectures of 1828; its author's long and useful life connects men still living with what seems a remote past. He was born in 1796, and there are still more than a dozen fellows of the College who may have sat in Comitia with him. He was admitted a fellow on 22 December 1826 and died in 1894. The copy of his book which I have read was presented by him to the Statistical (now Royal Statistical) Society in 1834 and contains corrections in his hand. Hawkins defines the province of Medical Statistics to be 'the application of numbers to illustrate the natural history of man in health and disease'. In his numerical statements he uses three indices; the ordinary crude death-rate—always expressed as one death in such or such a number—the 'probable life', i.e. the age to which half these born attain; the 'mean life', i.e. the average age at death. He was certainly aware that the age and sex constitution of a group affects the death-rate. Thus (op. cit. p. 20) he writes: 'In discussing the mortality of manufacturing towns or districts, it is just to remark that the small proportion is not always *real*; because a constant influx of *adults* is likely to render the number of deaths less considerable than that which could occur in a stationary population composed of all ages.' From the use of the term *stationary population* in this passage we may also, perhaps, infer that Hawkins knew the limitations of utility of such indices as mean age at death or *vie probable*, but I cannot fairly say that in making comparisons he calls attention to the dangers.

A modern treatise, such as that of Dr Hill, devotes a large space to methods of evaluating errors of sampling or, to speak loosely, the precautions to be taken when the observations are few in number and may not have been taken without bias. Some of the methods still employed had been invented by mathematicians before Hawkins's day, but he did not use them. On p. 32 we read: 'The annual mortality of Nice, though a small town, and enjoying a factitious reputation of salubrity, is 1 in 31; of Naples, is 1 in 28. Leghorn is more fortunate, and sinks to 1 in 35. We instance those places as being the frequent resort of invalids; but how astonishing is the superiority of England, when we compare with these even our great manufacturing towns, such as Manchester, 1 in 74; such as even Birmingham, 1 in 43; or even this overgrown metropolis, where the deaths are only 1 in 40.'

In the copy I have read, the sentence 'such as Manchester, 1 in 74' has been struck through, apparently by the author. But, even with this emendation, the comparison, to the glory of our country, is, well, tendentious.

Indeed, one must admit, however regretfully, that Hawkins's book is uncritical. He had been diligent and brought together numerical data from all parts of the world and was certainly one of the first physicians to advocate a serious study of hospital records, but one can hardly say that, as a statistician, he was better equipped or more efficient than Dr Short in 1750. But his modesty is disarming: 'I should be amply rewarded if the present humble essay should form a temporary repository of the most important of their labours; if it should become one of the early milestones on a road which is comparatively new, rugged as yet and uninviting to the distant traveller, but which gradually discloses the most interesting prospects, and will at length, if I do not deceive myself by premature anticipation, largely recompense the patient adventurer' (op. cit. p. vii).

According to Munk (*Roll*, **3**, 304) Hawkins was instrumental in obtaining the insertion in the first Registration Act of a column containing the names of the diseases or causes by which death was occasioned. 'At first the insertion was voluntary; it has since been made compulsory; and has produced important additions to medical and statistical science through the indefatigable labours of Dr W. Farr.'

So the name of Francis Bisset Hawkins deserves a place on the roll of benefactors to medical statistical science.

Eight years after the publication of Hawkins's Gulstonians there appeared, as Chapter IV of the fifth part of McCulloch's *Statistical Account of the British Empire* (**2**, 567–601, London, 1837), an article on 'Vital statistics; or the statistics of health, sickness, disease and death', the work of William Farr, then in his 30th year and still a general practitioner and free-lance medical journalist. It contains perhaps a quarter of the number of words in Hawkins's book and is not free from the quaint moralizing not always wholly relevant to the statistical theme which was characteristic of Farr, but it ranks not much below Graunt's 'Observations' as an original contribution to medical-statistical science.

Farr proposed to examine 'the mortality, the sickness, the endemics, the prevailing forms of disease, and the various ways in which, at all ages, its [The British Population's] successive generations perish'.

Slow as had been the progress of official statistics between 1662 and 1837, there had been progress. The four censuses of 1801–31 provided reasonably complete accounts of total populations. In 1821, information as to age was invited and eight-ninths of the population accepted the invitation. In 1831 the clergy were asked to return not merely totals of burials but burials classified by ages for the 18 years ending in 1830. These latter returns were incomplete, but it was possible for a lesser man than Farr to approximate to a statement of rates of mortality at ages at least for the period centring on 1821. To Farr's annoyance, the census takers of 1831 did not ask for the ages of the enumerated, contenting themselves with an enumeration of males under and over 20 years of age. The data for computing mortality rates were particularly defective for towns, but a few instances of quite good voluntary enumerations, e.g. for Carlisle and Glasgow, were available.

In handling national rates of mortality at ages, Farr's article does not display any conspicuous originality; he, quite properly, used the work of predecessors and he does not comment on the defects of the data. He does, however, call attention to particular rates of mortality, for instance, those of the troops, in an emphatic way. 'By the subjoined table of the mortality of the British army it will be seen that the soldier, in the prime of his physical powers, is rendered more liable to death every step he takes from his native climate, till at last the man of 28 years is subject, in the West Indies, to the same mortality as the man of 80 remaining in Britain.' According to his table, the average strength of British troops in Jamaica and Honduras between 1810 and 1828 was 2528; in the year of least mortality the rate 47 per 1000, the average 113 and the maximum 472! In the United Kingdom the average rate was 15 per 1000.

The most original part of Farr's essay is his treatment of sickness. Here national statistics were not available; more than 70 years were to pass before any nation-wide data were collected, and the statistics of morbidity still lag behind those of mortality. All Farr had were some data of benefit societies and returns relating to workers in the Royal Dockyards and employees of the East India Company. He begins by stating that in manhood for every death we may reckon two persons constantly sick. It is not quite clear how he reached this ratio, but probably from a comparison of the mortality rates for 1815–30 shown in a table on p. 568 of his article with some theoretical rates deduced by Edmonds for Friendly Societies (op. cit. p. 574). One has:

Age	Sickness rate per 1000	Mortality rate per 1000
20–30	17·2	10·1
30–40	23·0	11·4
40–50	31·0	14·9
50–60	45·1	23·4
60–70	93·6	45·3

Taking the general rate of mortality to be 21·3 per 1000 and the population of England and Wales to be 14,000,000, he concludes that 600,000 persons are constantly sick and that the productive power of the community is reduced by one-seventeenth part (he has made allowance for attendance on the sick). He works out from the limited data available the relation between sick-time and age and concludes that it increases in geometrical progression up to the age of 50. He asks how much sickness exists among the labourers of the country independently of those definitely incapacitated by disease. Data for the Royal Dockyards lead him to conclude that 2% are constantly kept at home by illness.

In the last section of his article, Farr considers particular diseases. An instance of his acumen is to be seen in his criticism of the view (held in 1837 as in 1937) that insanity was on the increase. He pertinently remarks that if the less barbaric treatment of lunatics diminished the mortality rate a higher proportion of enumerated lunatics would be perfectly consistent with a steady rate of morbidity.

His data for rates of mortality by causes were scanty. For London over a long period he had causes of death in age groups and, from an estimate of total mortality in age groups, could pass back to rates at ages by causes. Heysham's Carlisle data were medically and statistically more precise but limited to one not large town. The data of the Equitable Assurance Society were numerous but, as, of course, Farr knew and emphasized, related to a select class of the population.

Some of his general conclusions were as follows:

It has been shown that external agents have as great an influence on the frequency of sickness as on its fatality; the obvious corollary is, that man has as much power to prevent as to cure disease. That prevention is better than cure, is a proverb; that it is as easy, the facts we had advanced establish. Yet medical men, the guardians of public health, never have their attention called to the prevention of sickness; it forms no part of their education. To promote health is apparently contrary to their interests: the public do not seek the shield of medical art against disease, nor call the surgeon, till the arrows of death already rankle in the veins. This may be corrected by modifying the present system of medical education, and the manner of remunerating medical men.

Public health may be promoted by placing the medical institutions of the country on a liberal scientific basis; by medical societies co-operating to collect statistical observations; and by medical writers renouncing the notion that a science can be founded upon the limited experience of an individual. Practical medicine cannot be taught in books; the science of medicine cannot be acquired in the sick room. The healing art may likewise be promoted by encouraging post-mortem examinations of diseased parts; without which it is impossible to keep up in the body of the medical profession a clear knowledge of the internal change indicated by symptoms during life. The practitioner who never opens a dead body must commit innumerable, and sometimes fatal, errors (op. cit. p. 601).

Farr's article closes the epoch Graunt's book opened. The seventeenth-century pioneer did not live to see the ground he broke bear a crop. The high gods used Farr better; he lived to create the best official vital-statistics of the world. It is true that the lessons he taught were learned but slowly, either by the public or the faculty. The *Annual Reports* of the Registrar-General will not be found among the frequently consulted volumes on the shelves of Fellows of the College of Physicians. But something has been learned. The moral truism that human vanity is a deadly sin, now exemplified on a world-wide scale, is illustrated on the humbler scale of those topics which have been my life's work and the subject of these lectures. The distrust of 'mathematical' methods which is still general in our profession is not primarily due to the mere intellectual difficulty of learning 'mathematical' methods; much that all medical students must learn is at least as difficult.

The roots are deeper. They begin with the exaggerated claims of the iatro-mathematicians of the late seventeenth and early eighteenth centuries. The personal popularity of such men as Freind and Jurin did not conceal the fact that pathology and clinical medicine reduced to mechanical and quantitative theorems, and 'proofs' were of not much greater value in the treatment of sick men than skill in playing chess to the commander of an army. It is arguable that a talent for playing chess might, other things equal, be of advantage to a military strategist (Napoleon Bonaparte was very fond of chess and played so badly that it was difficult for his staff to avoid winning), but other things are not equal. In later times, when the intellectual prestige of mathematical science had grown enormously, it was observed that such an Admirable Crichton as our Thomas Young was inferior as a practical physician to many fellows of lesser fame. In our generation when the professional mathematicians who, 50 years ago, rather despised mere statistics, have increasingly devoted themselves to the improvement of the general theory, the complexity of statistical investigations has done little to attract the amateur, and intellectual modesty has not been the most conspicuous virtue of statistical authors. Perhaps, too, it is not easy for an experienced physician 'to renounce the notion that a science can be founded upon the limited experience of an individual'.

The moral I should draw from the history of medical statistics is that the intellectual courage of an amateur often succeeds where erudition fails. While even the purest of mathematicians would not claim that statistics is only a branch of mathematics, the hardiest contemner of algebra would admit that a training in mathematical method is an advantage to the practical statistician. The mathematician would surely agree that a knowledge of the material subjected to analysis was valuable, even if not so essential as a 'practical' man would claim.

Judged by contemporary intellectual standards, neither Graunt nor Farr was a mathematician; Graunt had no medical training, Farr's clinical experience was meagre. In respect neither of method nor subject-matter was either man an expert. But they both had intellectual curiosity and courage: one may say, if one pleases, the spurious courage of the man who is brave because he does not know what the dangers are. But, as Gilbert Chesterton once said, 'There is no real hope that has not once been a forlorn hope.' In graver matters than medical statistics and more than once in our national history salvation has been wrought by courageous amateurs who acted while professionals doubted.

Those who cannot disclaim a professional status in statistics, whether officials or professors, may learn a lesson from history. It is conveyed in the four words: *maxima debetur puero reverentia*, construing *puer* by amateur or beginner or enthusiast. It is weary work to read statistical 'proofs' of this or that aetiological theory of cancer, or proposals for this or that impossible statistical investigation. But it is treachery to science to rebuff any genuinely inquisitive person; the discovery of another Graunt in a shop or another Farr in the surgery of a general practitioner would repay the life-long boredom of all extant civil servants and professors of statistics.